Creating Successful Dementia Care Settings

Volume 4

Enhancing Identity and Sense of Home

The complete set of books in
Creating Successful Dementia Care Settings
includes

Volume 1: **Understanding the Environment Through Aging Senses**
Volume 2: **Maximizing Cognitive and Functional Abilities**
Volume 3: **Minimizing Disruptive Behaviors**
Volume 4: **Enhancing Identity and Sense of Home**

Training videos for
Creating Successful Dementia Care Settings
include

Maximizing Cognitive and Functional Abilities (companion to Volume 2)
Minimizing Disruptive Behaviors (companion to Volume 3)
Enhancing Self and Sense of Home (companion to Volume 4)
(See ordering information at end of book.)

Creating Successful Dementia Care Settings

Developed by Margaret P. Calkins, M.Arch., Ph.D.

Volume 4
Enhancing Identity and Sense of Home

Volume Authors
John P. Marsden, M.Arch., Ph.D.,
Sherylyn H. Briller, Ph.D.,
Margaret P. Calkins, M.Arch., Ph.D.,
and Mark A. Proffitt, M.Arch.

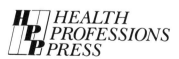
HEALTH PROFESSIONS PRESS

Baltimore • London • Winnipeg • Sydney

Health Professions Press, Inc.
Post Office Box 10624
Baltimore, Maryland 21285-0624

www.healthpropress.com

Typeset by Barton Matheson Willse & Worthington, Baltimore, Maryland.
Printed in the United States of America by Versa Press, Inc., East Peoria, Illinois.
Interior illustrations by David Fedan.

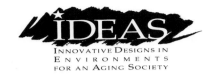

Margaret P. Calkins, M.Arch., Ph.D., is president of I.D.E.A.S. (Innovative Designs in Environments for an Aging Society), Inc., a consultation, education, and research firm dedicated to exploring the therapeutic potential of the environment as it relates to older adults who are frail and impaired. I.D.E.A.S., Inc., is based in Kirtland, Ohio.

The case examples in this book series are based on the authors' actual experiences. In all instances, names and identifying details have been changed to protect confidentiality.

Library of Congress Cataloging-in-Publication Data

Calkins, Margaret P.
　　Creating successful dementia care settings / developed by Margaret P. Calkins.
　　　　p.　　cm.
　　Includes bibliographical references and index.
　　Contents: Vol. 1. Understanding the environment through aging senses—v. 2. Maximizing cognitive and functional abilities—v. 3. Minimizing disruptive behaviors—v. 4. Enhancing identity and sense of home.
　　　　ISBN 1-878812-72-6 (v. 1)—ISBN 1-878812-73-4 (v. 2)—ISBN 1-878812-74-2 (v. 3)—ISBN 1-878812-75-0 (v. 4)
　　　　1. Dementia—Patients—Care.　2. Dementia—Patients—Long-term care.　3. Health facilities—Administration.　I. Title.

RC521.C35 2001
362.1′9683—dc21　　　　　　　　　　　　　　　　　　　　　　　2001039141

British Cataloguing in Publication Data are available from the British Library.

Series Contents

Volume 2

Volume 3

Volume 4

About the Authors

Margaret P. Calkins, M.Arch., Ph.D., is President of I.D.E.A.S. Inc. (Innovative Designs in Environments for an Aging Society), a consultation, education, and research firm dedicated to exploring the therapeutic potential of the environment—social and organizational as well as physical—particularly as it relates to older adults who are frail and impaired. She is also Senior Fellow Emeritus of the Institute on Aging and Environment at the University of Wisconsin-Milwaukee.

Dr. Calkins holds degrees in both psychology and architecture. A member of several national organizations and panels that focus on issues of care for older adults with cognitive impairment, she speaks frequently at conferences nationally and internationally. She has published extensively, and her book *Design for Dementia: Planning Environments for the Elderly and the Confused* (National Health Publication, 1998) was the first comprehensive design guide for special care units for people with dementia.

Dr. Calkins is Director and a founding member of SAGE (Society for the Advancement of Gerontological Environments), and has been a juror for numerous design competitions.

Sherylyn H. Briller, Ph.D., is Assistant Professor of Anthropology at Wayne State University. She is a medical anthropologist who specializes in aging research. Dr. Briller received her master's and doctorate degrees and a graduate certificate in gerontology from Case Western Reserve University. She has been actively involved in the field of aging for more than a decade, both domestically and abroad. Her diverse career has included working as an activities coordinator in a skilled nursing facility, a program director at a community senior center, and a gerontological researcher in the United States of America and Asia. Her long-term care expertise includes philosophy/model of care, staff training, activity programming, and ethnic/cultural issues relating to aging. She has consulted, published, and given presentations to numerous audiences including policy makers, researchers, administrators, direct caregivers, and consumers.

John P. Marsden, M.Arch., Ph.D., is an assistant professor in the College of Design, Construction and Planning and a core faculty member of the Institute on Aging at the University of Florida. He holds degrees in architecture from Carnegie Mellon University, the University of Arizona, and the University of Michigan. Dr. Marsden has worked for several architecture firms, was an associate at I.D.E.A.S., Inc., and has consulted with designers and long-term care administrators. He is a frequent speaker at gerontology and environmental design conferences and served as a juror for the 1999 Best of Seniors' Housing Awards, sponsored by the National Council on Seniors' Housing, a division of the National Association of Home Builders.

Kristin Perez, OTR/L, received her bachelor's degree in gerontology from Bowling Green State University and a certificate in occupational therapy from Cleveland State University. Ms. Perez has experience in direct care, programming, management, and research in dementia care settings. She has assisted older adults in maximizing their level of independence and life satisfaction in assisted living, nursing facility, adult day services, and hospital settings. Ms. Perez has been actively involved in numerous research projects addressing dementia care practices and environments, including project management. She has also provided consultation to long-term care facilities regarding dementia care practices and environmental influences.

Mark A. Proffitt, M.Arch., is an architectural researcher with Dorsky Hodgson + Partners, an architectural firm that specializes in designs for older adults. His primary responsibilities include post-occupancy evaluations of completed projects and the programming protocol for the elderly design studio. He strongly believes that good design must build on research. Mr. Proffitt received his master's degree in architecture from the University of Wisconsin–Milwaukee, where he was a fellow with the Institute on Aging and Environment. After receiving his degree, he served as a facilities architect and manager for a developer of retirement communities. Mr. Proffitt has also co-authored a book on the creation and evaluation of an innovative health center and has spoken at several industry-related conferences.

Acknowledgments

Creative endeavors are nurtured to fruition by the ideas and efforts of myriad people at every step of a process. While the original conceptualization for the project was spearheaded by Maggie Calkins, with input from Jerry Weisman, this was very much a team project. All of the authors' talents and contributions were integral and critical to the evolution of the larger project from which these volumes are drawn. In addition, Eileen Lipstreuer, Chari Weber, and Rebecca Meehan deserve as much credit for their contributions to the project as the names that appear on the title pages of these volumes. The videos that accompany these volumes are a direct result of their industriousness. Thanks also to Jesse Epstein, of Cinecraft, and David Litz, the videographer, and to David Fedan for his charming illustrations.

Much of the project was funded by the National Institute on Aging (grant R44 AG12311) and enthusiastically supported and championed by Marcia Ory. We were also fortunate to have a team of nationally recognized experts whose input—both conceptual and practical—was invaluable. We extend our gratitude to Powell Lawton, Jerry Weisman, Phil Sloane, Joe Foley, Susan Gilster, Kitty Buckwalter, Jeanne Teresi, Doug Holmes, and Sheryl Zimmerman. Peter Whitehouse, Elisabeth Koss, Clive Gilmore, and Monte Levinson shared their keen intellect and significant insight with us as we started this project. During the most stressful periods of the project, Cassie and Ted always seemed to come to our rescue.

We would like to thank the numerous individuals whose publications and conference presentations enriched our understanding of the complex nature of dementia, and provided myriad ideas for creative solutions to difficult challenges. We also appreciate the endless hours of listening and thoughtful contributions of the many family, friends, and colleagues who helped out in so many ways as the project evolved over 4 years. To the numerous facility staff and administrators who listened to, read, questioned, and critiqued our efforts and dialogued with us about them, it was for you that we embarked on this voyage. We are pleased to share what we have learned with you.

Preface

All too often, we see well-intentioned caregivers unnecessarily limit or down-play the potential remaining abilities of the older adults with dementia for whom they care. Caregivers seem to assume that because a person has demen-tia, every behavior and every expression of anxiety, fear, or anger is a direct consequence of the dementing illness. And, because dementia impairs care recipients' cognitive abilities, many caregivers believe that they have the right and the responsibility to make all decisions for those they care for.

It has been the authors' experience that the factors that affect the behav-ior of residents with dementia are complex. Our approach to understanding their behavior focuses on the person, on his or her typical needs and desires, on the limitations imposed by age-related changes, and on the effects of aspects of the environment.

Our fundamental philosophy is that we must first consider those in our care as people, who have many of the same needs, desires, and wishes as any-one else. To lose the ability to make decisions that affect virtually every aspect of living is devastating. To have that ability further eroded by care providers and care settings that eliminate almost every opportunity for choice and con-trol is unacceptable.

It is the authors' hope that in using the information contained within *Creating Successful Dementia Care Settings*, facilities will create meaningful care settings by educating and sensitizing staff and by making full use of the envi-ronmental resources available to them.

User's Guide

The authors' goal in writing this four-volume series was to create an easy-to-use reference to help care providers understand and more appropriately manage, through the environment, the broad array of behaviors and changing abilities that occur with dementia. One must first recognize the importance of accommodating the basic needs of all people, and then one must consider that most people with dementia are older and, therefore, experience the world through sensory modalities that are changing or that have been altered by aging. Vision, hearing, touch, taste, and smell all change with age, and sensory changes often affect behavior. For example, it may not be dementia but simply poor vision that hinders a person's ability to read signs or an activity calendar. Volume 1, *Understanding the Environment Through Aging Senses* helps caregivers to be more sensitive to how these sensory changes can affect a person's basic functioning.

Only after the needs of the resident as a person like anyone else and as an older person with changing sensory experiences have been acknowledged can one consider the unique needs of the individual as an older person with dementia. There is no denying that the neuropathological changes that occur in the brain of a person with dementia affect his or her ability to perceive, make sense of, and operate effectively in the surrounding environment. Basic tasks, such as dressing and eating, that once were easy become increasingly difficult. The inability to interpret what someone is saying, to identify faces or objects, or to understand his or her current location can easily lead to fear and resistance to care. Volumes 2 and 3, *Maximizing Cognitive and Functional Abilities* and *Minimizing Disruptive Behaviors*, respectively, focus on these issues.

Enhancing Identity and Sense of Home, Volume 4, addresses issues that are primarily related to basic human needs such as privacy, autonomy, identity, and personal space. Much of the information is appropriate not only for people with dementia but also for cognitively alert individuals in long-term care settings.

The more that you, as a caregiver, understand all of the factors that affect the person or people whose care is entrusted to you, the better able you are to see the world as they do. Thus, the beginning of each chapter in all of the volumes presents the individual topic from the residents' perspective, including contributing factors and influences on specific behaviors or issues. In addition, these sections offer ideas for assessing problems and implementing interventions. This level of information is particularly useful for staff members who manage and/or train direct care staff. The authors hope that this information will broaden staff's knowledge on the topic and that they will pass the information along to others who care for residents.

The residents' perspective section is followed by "What Staff Can Do," which provides information on social interactions between staff and residents and ideas for structured and spontaneous activities on the unit. Some interventions focus on teaching direct care staff to take a different approach to particular situations, whereas other interventions are provided for staff who plan structured activities and programs.

The third main section of each chapter, "What the Environment Can Do," offers suggestions for modifications or changes that can be made to the physical environment so that your facility becomes more supportive of the residents, particularly those with dementia. Many of the suggested changes cost nothing and involve only a different use of the environment or a small modification using materials you probably already have on hand. Other changes are low in cost, requiring the purchase of a few additional products or materials. Finally, if your facility is able to upgrade or replace some of its furnishings or equipment, we have provided practical advice in "What the Environment Can Do" on what to consider when purchasing a product. Many of the modifications suggested in this section explain how these modifications benefit the residents and the staff who care for them.

The final section of each chapter, "Where to Find Products," lists specific manufacturers and distributors of the products mentioned in the text. There is some repetition in these sections across the four volumes so that you do not have to refer to a separate volume for the information. Many of the manufacturers and catalogs also carry more products than those highlighted in our lists. This section is followed by a summary sheet, which boils down the chapter text into an easy-to-remember, quick overview. We have also provided an area for you to make notes about your own staff and facility. Managerial staff may wish to use the summary sheets as handouts to accompany direct care staff training, or to post them by the time clock or nurses' station or include them in staff's pay envelopes. All staff, including business office, social services, dietary, and housekeeping, may appreciate this quick overview of issues because they likely interact with residents daily.

At the conclusion of each volume, a detailed bibliography and suggested readings help you learn more about issues in the individual volumes. The Behavior Tracking Form and Sensory Stimulation Assessment appendixes appear at the end of Volume 3. Staff can use these forms to examine the occurrence of behaviors and aspects of the environment more closely. Each blank form is accompanied by explanatory information and a sample completed form. Volume 4 includes three appendixes, all designed to help residents feel more at home in the facility and to protect their safety.

In addition to the four volumes, there are three videotapes that relate to Volumes 2–4. They were designed to be staff education resources and provide an additional way of helping all staff learn how to create successful dementia care settings (see ordering information at the end of each volume).

We at I.D.E.A.S., Inc., wish you success in developing a high-quality environment for caregiving. It is our hope that facilities will use this information to create meaningful dementia care settings by educating and sensitizing staff. If you are having a hard time determining which aspects of your care setting most need to be changed or modified, we hope that you will contact us directly (440-256-1880 or info@IDEASconsultingInc.com).

1

Overview of Home-Based Philosophy of Care

Because this volume is dedicated to identity and sense of home, many of the recommendations found throughout reflect a home-based philosophy. Although a home-based philosophy is not the only appropriate model of care, this model is emphasized because it is one that many long-term care facilities attempt to achieve. Unfortunately, the vast majority of these facilities seem to be unclear about what a home-based philosophy really entails, and they often mix different philosophies without realizing it. Others may have a mission statement, but it is often written in such general terms, sometimes for marketing purposes only, that it does not provide

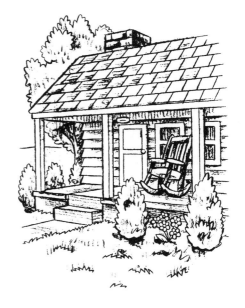

the basis for structuring the care setting. In addition, there are few studies that deal with this topic in any detail. The Alzheimer's Association's *Key Elements of Dementia Care* (1997) lists some of the elements that should be included in a facility's mission statement (e.g., program philosophy, whom the program serves, the approach to care, program location). However, these are largely process-oriented recommendations and do not provide content-based information.

This section offers a brief overview of a home-based philosophy as well as some of the other philosophies that are typically incorporated within care settings. By clearly defining and differentiating several philosophies, a facility will be able to define its model of care more clearly, and create care and service plans that accurately reflect that model. Thus, it is important for facilities to review their mission statement—if they have one—and determine whether it reflects their current goals and whether their care practices support that mission. The mission statement, or philosophy, is one of the most important components of a care setting and should be the foundation on which all care decisions are made. It can drive how the policies are written, what the approach to care is, how staff are trained, how staff should interact with residents, how the daily program is organized, and how the environment should be structured.

MODELS OF CARE

Medical Model

The medical model has its roots in the development and evaluation of nursing facilities. When nursing facilities first were authorized by the federal government under the Hill-Burton Act of 1954, they were viewed as subacute hospitals for people with chronic conditions. Thus, many of the codes and regulations that affected nursing facilities were drawn directly from hospital codes, and were primarily medically based. It was also expected that many of the residents would spend the vast majority of their days in bed, passively receiving care provided by professionals.

In the medical model of care, it is primarily the diagnosis—or, frequently, diagnoses—of the patient that drive the plan of care, and medical care takes priority over program aspects that support the social or psychological needs of the patient. For instance, medications, even those that do not require administration at specific times, are delivered at the convenience of the nurse. When patients are engaged in an activity, either the activity is interrupted while the medications are passed to several patients or one patient is pulled out of the program to be given his or her medications. In addition, programs and activities tend to be designed primarily to keep people occupied for periods of time, and thus often are designed for large numbers of residents. Meals tend to be highly structured: Typically, food is plated in the kitchen and served on trays to control portion size, and meals occur at specific times designed to balance the amount of time between them. In general, all residents are required to be seated at all meals, including those who are on liquid diets. At night, all residents are checked on once or twice (even those who routinely sleep through the night uninterrupted) on the presumption that there might be a change in status or that a resident might need assistance but not be able to ask for it.

Many of these care practices are written into the state or federal regulatory system, and thus are required for virtually all nursing facilities. There are good and valid reasons for all of these regulations, either in terms of expected health benefits or in terms of regulating the quality of care and ensuring that at least minimal standards are met. However, the primary emphasis clearly is on treating the medical needs of the residents. Although this may be appropriate for many people who reside in nursing facilities, it is not always suitable for individuals with early- or moderate-stage dementia.

Residential Model

Interest has developed in creating a model of care that is not as exclusively focused on the medical condition of the resident. The impetus for this model was an increased recognition of the needs of people with Alzheimer's disease and related dementias. Many individuals with dementia are active and quite healthy physically, and often they do not fall into the category of residents that nursing facilities were originally designed to serve. Individuals with dementia, who are not likely to spend much time each day in their rooms in bed, may find group activities overstimulating and often resist receiving care, either because they think they do not need it or because they do not understand what is being done to them. (Volume 3 covers this topic in more detail.) Historically, the main method of coping with these care challenges was to restrain residents, either physically or chemically, so they would fit better within the structure of the medical model. By the mid-1980s, it became apparent that this was not an appropriate way to provide care for residents of long-term care facilities.

As a result, the residential model began to evolve. Based on the recognition that people with dementia have a harder time learning new information, it was hypothesized that a setting that was more familiar might enable them to function better. It was thought that the program and physical design of long-term care facilities should emulate the homes in which most people with dementia would have lived in the community. The challenges, however, have been substantial—particularly in nursing facilities. Despite changes in philosophy, codes and regulations still can be restrictive. As a result, many of the innovations in dementia care settings are found typically in assisted living or residential care settings. The regulations for these building types are not nearly as strict as they are for nursing facilities.

Regardless of the setting, a primary goal of the residential model is to maintain as much continuity with each resident's past as possible. The day is structured as it might have been at home. This means there might be more flexible times for meals. For instance, a hot breakfast might be served from 7:00 A.M. to 8:30 A.M., and a continental breakfast might be available both earlier and later for those who would like to choose when they want to rise. Lunch might be offered from 11:30 A.M. to 1:00 P.M. so that residents who choose not to have breakfast can eat an earlier lunch. Dinner also might be offered at various times. Of course, residents also should be given some choice in what is served (Zgola & Bordillon, 2001). Emphasis in activities is placed on enabling residents to continue to engage in the types of things they did at home, which might include domestic chores related to meal preparation and cleanup and household maintenance (from dusting and cleaning to raking leaves or hanging laundry), or social activities outside the home (bridge club, weekly bingo, or meeting friends at the local bar to watch a Monday night football game). In addition, the delivery of medication usually does not conflict with the activity program. Although there are always exceptions—times when a medication must be administered—the regular scheduling of medical services is designed so that it does not conflict with or take precedence over the other aspects of the program.

To develop programs that meet each resident's individual needs, facility staff must get to know the residents well. Specific strategies for doing so are provided throughout this volume. However, developing an activities program that is geared toward different functional and cognitive levels of residents is one of the more significant challenges to providing a residential model. A resident who has severe cognitive impairment may not be able to participate in baking cookies or muffins as actively as a resident with less impairment, but he or she can still participate if the activity is structured in small steps. Even residents with the most severe impairments can participate vicariously by smelling the aroma of baking cookies. We have no way of knowing, however, whether these types of aroma cues can help a resident make connections to earlier times when he or she cannot express these connections outwardly.

Of all of the models of care, the residential model has the strongest relationship to a specific set of environmental elements. For example, there is a certain layout or arrangement of spaces that is common to virtually all houses—the front door leads into the more public and formal areas of the house, and the back door typically leads into the kitchen or possibly a casual family room. (This is covered in more detail in Chapter 6 later in this volume.) Unfortunately, it is difficult, if not impossible, to try to create this arrangement of spaces within existing long-term care settings. However, there are other ways to reflect a residential model through physical features. For instance, because of the emphasis on continuity of self, the facility can strongly encourage residents to bring some of their own furniture, and not just for their bedrooms. Most people put many of their most cherished and personally significant possessions in the public areas of their homes, such as the living room and dining room. To achieve a residential model requires that residents feel that the whole care unit, not just their bedrooms, is their home.

Finally, there are ways in which the relationship between caregivers and those receiving care can be structured to be residential-like. For instance, having staff wear street clothes instead of uniforms can suggest that they are more like surrogate family caregivers than paid professional staff. Another way to break down the traditional hierarchy of roles is for staff to eat meals with the residents, just the way family caregivers do. All aspects of the program should try to reflect what life was like at home before relocating to the long-term care setting.

Hospitality Model

Another model of care that is referred to throughout this volume is similar in some ways to the residential model but different in a number of fundamental ways. The advances in medical care in the 20th century have resulted in a significant number of healthier older individuals. Coupled with a healthy, growing economy, many older individuals also have significant financial resources at their command. As a result, there has been tremendous growth in the number of retirement communities that are designed to support the lifestyles and leisure activities of well-to-do retirees. Organizations have responded to this potentially lucrative market by developing service-oriented supportive living settings. These are most prevalent in continuing care retirement communities but increasingly are spreading to assisted living and even a few licensed nursing facilities. They also can be seen in a growing number of dementia-specific care settings. This model is referred to as the *hospitality* or *spa model.*

In the hospitality model, the individuals served are often referred to as *customers* and may include family members as well as the residents themselves. The overarching philosophy is to give customers what they want. Thus, residents are catered to more than they would be in the residential model. For instance, residents are more likely to have choices of entrees at meals and be served restaurant-style by the staff. Theme evenings (e.g., Hawaiian night) provide a break in the routine. Residents are not expected to help with meal preparation, nor are they encouraged to clean or dust their rooms. Similarly, activities are designed to entertain the residents. In most cases, residents can choose among multiple, simultaneous activities, ideally geared toward different interests and different cognitive and functional skills. For instance, one group of residents might gather each morning to go over the newspaper, while another resident might be encouraged to take his or her morning walk, and still another might be shown a travel or animal-oriented video.

Facilities that follow a hospitality model resemble fine hotels or resorts. Grand two-storied lobbies, elegantly decorated dining rooms, and cathedral ceilings are common. Finish materials (wall coverings, window treatments, and flooring) also tend to be more formal than what most people have in their homes. These facilities may also have a concierge desk instead of a reception or staff station.

CONCLUSION

There is no "correct" or "best" philosophy for all care settings. The choice of an appropriate philosophy depends on many factors, including the level of care, the acuity levels of the residents, the tenets of the organization, and the sociocultural background of both residents and staff. However, by clearly defining and differentiating several philosophies, the facility can define its model of care more clearly, and can create care and service plans that accurately reflect that model. Every staff member should be aware of and buy into the philosophy, and families also should know the philosophy of the facility or dementia program. In other words, everyone should have similar knowledge of and expectations about how care in the setting is structured. For instance, if a facility chooses to implement a residential or homelike model of care, then residents probably would expect to see or participate in familiar domestic activities such as helping with the meal service, rather than gross motor exercises such as parachute ball games that are more typical of a medical or rehabilitative approach.

2
Personalization

What makes people interesting is that they all are different. As unique individuals, people have specific tastes, preferences, and identities. This is noticeable when you look at the clothes, makeup, and hairstyles people wear or the cars they drive. For instance, some people may like to drive trucks; others may prefer sedans or may like riding on motorcycles. Individuality is also noticeable when you look at the homes people choose and the changes they make to those homes through additions, decoration, or furniture arrangements. For example, some people may decide to display pink flamingos on their front lawns, whereas others pre-

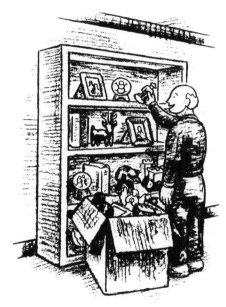

fer to plant flowers instead. Some may, after a few years, refinish hardwood floors in their living rooms to show off a rug passed down by a grandparent, and others may prefer to stick with the warmth of wall-to-wall carpeting. When people change their environments to suit their tastes and to express their uniqueness or individuality, they are engaging in personalization. The reasons why personalization is important are many, ranging from opportunities for expressing the self and understanding the self to marking a home as one's own.

EXPRESSING THE SELF

When Lori and Tim returned home last night, their house was burning and the fire was out of control. Photographs, family treasures, clothes, mementos, and furniture were lost in the fire. Losing these items was heart wrenching to Lori and Tim because these items were a part of their lives and their past. They told a story about Lori and Tim, and were a way to show others who they were as individuals. Although they still have their selves, representing this externally without their possessions would be difficult.

Lori and Tim started house hunting after the fire. They noticed that many of the houses in the neighborhood where they were looking appeared similar. This made it difficult for them to tell a story about themselves once again. After selecting a house and moving in, they set about personalizing the inside and outside of the new home to differentiate it from others in the neighborhood and to express themselves as unique individuals (Cooper, 1974). They painted the outside of the house blue in contrast to the many white homes located on their street, and they added decorative features such as window shutters. They also replaced the front door, outside lights, and mailbox and changed the landscaping by adding flowers, shrubs, wood chips, and rocks. Inside the house, they painted the walls, selected and arranged furniture, installed curtains, hung pictures, and set out knickknacks and plants.

When we make changes to the outside of our houses as Lori and Tim did, we are expressing the selves that we wish to show others, such as neighbors and acquaintances. This image may or may not be a true representation of the self, but it is one that we have chosen and over which we have control. Within our houses, we may make changes that express the self we wish to share with the people we invite inside, such as family members and close friends. We may select from different furniture styles, arrange those furnishings, install curtains or blinds, display meaningful objects, choose paint colors or wallpaper, hang pictures and artwork, and purchase a variety of plants. For example, some people buy one hard-to-kill plant and others express their love of nature and gardening by filling the house with many plants. These choices help us to express what is important to us. In the process, we actually project something of ourselves onto the physical environment. Imagine how frustrating it would be if you were not able to make these types of changes. Some apartment buildings, for example, force tenants to follow rules that forbid them to change the color of the carpeting or to put nail holes in the walls to hang pictures.

UNDERSTANDING THE SELF

Have you ever noticed that most of the changes you made to your house or your parents made to their house occurred first when children were born and then again when the children left home? For example, you may have added furniture after a child was born and later turned a playroom into a television-viewing room after your youngest child married. You also may have noticed that one friend in particular always spends a great deal of time taking care of his or her home and garden—maintaining and renewing it—as if to convey loving respect, whereas another friend may have made few changes over the years after settling in, as if to suggest contentment and stability. In other words, personalization can reflect where you are in your life and how you feel about yourself. Personalizing can lead you to a greater understanding of yourself (Cooper, 1974).

In contrast, choosing not to personalize shows less of the self externally but can also reveal where you are in your life and how you feel about things. For example, when you rent an apartment on a temporary basis, you might not bother displaying knickknacks or hanging pictures on walls. Even though you own these objects, you might choose to keep them packed in boxes because you are not interested in putting down roots right now. (The same may hold true for residents of long-term care facilities, who believe they will eventually go home or are, as some say, "just waiting to die.") In other instances, you might not have the time or the money to make changes to a house. A single working mother might be busy taking care of her children and managing her job. Personalization may be a lower priority in her life at such a time.

MARKING A TERRITORY AS YOUR OWN

Were you to look around your neighborhood, you would probably find at least one house surrounded by a fence or shrubs. If you were to walk onto the property toward the house, you might find a nameplate on the front door. The occupant probably used the fence and nameplate deliberately not only to reflect his or her identity but also to state "this is my area." This type of personalization "allows a person to lay claim to an area" that is the individual's own "and have control over it" (Calkins, 1988, p. 25) (see Chapter 5 for additional information). In other words, if people stake out an area, then they must be able to convey this to others, and personalization is an effective way to accomplish it.

HOW PERSONALIZATION
CHANGES WITH AGE AND RELOCATION

Older people sometimes mention that they are shocked by their appearance in the mirror. They may say that they feel like the same person they have always been, yet they look different. With aging, older adults often experience many significant losses, including physical changes in appearance as well as retirement and the death of loved ones, that can erode their sense of self. As a result, older people may try to do what they can to help them recognize their many selves. For example, many older people use cosmetics and hair dyes to try to stay young looking. Some older adults display a retirement plaque or hang a company jacket in a prominent location in their home because work was such a significant part of their identity. Thus, personalizing an environment may help older adults to preserve their self or keep it intact (Hummon, 1989; Marsden, 1993).

Preserving the Self

During a visit to his grandparents' house, Mark notices that his grandmother has a lot of possessions, some of which are not to his taste or are dated. In particular, his grandmother has a chair that Mark's grandfather sat in every night to read the newspaper, watch television, and smoke his pipe. The fabric is outdated and worn along the arm supports, and the seat cushion still smells slightly of pipe smoke. Mark suggests making room in the house by putting the chair in the trash. His grandmother strongly objects, explaining that this chair is special and meaningful because it reminds her of Mark's grandfather, who has been deceased for a few years. Even though she can afford a new chair, she wants this one.

Possessions may be meaningful for many reasons. First, they are connections to an individual's historical past. Mark's grandmother's chair is a concrete object that is associated with his grandfather and certain activities such as reading the newspaper. Although some may believe that his grandmother is living in the past by keeping this chair, an alternative view is that she is actually using the past to affirm her present self (Tobin, 1996) and to retain continuity of that self. In addition, certain objects, unlike the aging self, do not change much over time and thus help to preserve coherence of the self.

In particular, research has shown that photographs serve this purpose and are the most cherished possessions of older adults (Csikszentmihalyi & Rochberg-Halton, 1981).

Second, possessions may be meaningful because they are a way to span across past generations. Objects may have been handed down to older adults by parents or other close family members. Often, these possessions are associated with certain people or with a story. Possessions also can be used to link to future generations. Older people may choose to bequeath certain objects following their deaths or may pass on certain items during their lifetimes. Often, this is a way for older individuals to preserve and share the self with generations to come. Items that often are used to span past and future generations include genealogical records, photographs, jewelry, art, and furniture as well as religious objects such as bibles, prayer books, crucifixes, or menorahs (Tobin, 1996).

Third, possessions can evoke memories. Older adults who are experiencing decreases in visual acuity may not need to see familiar possessions well for those possessions to evoke memories. These memories often are tied to special relationships the older person may have had with others as well as to specific life events. For example, a cookbook given to an older woman by her mother on a birthday may remind her of her mother as well as the many times they spent together cooking, experimenting with new dishes, and exchanging recipes. This can certainly be a comforting and pleasurable experience. Although the reminiscing may or may not be accurate, the memory triggered is important because it affirms the self and reminds older people of their identities.

Relocation

In addition to the physical and social losses that older people may face as a result of aging, they also may have to deal with the loss of a home if it becomes necessary for them to relocate to a long-term care setting. The majority of older adults associate home with a privately owned single-family house. Throughout life, they have been able to display personal items, decorate walls, and arrange furniture freely within the house, as well as select exterior paint colors and garden outside. Most older people also have spent a great deal of time and energy creating an identity that is expressed and preserved by their houses. In other words, many older people feel that their home is who they are.

When older adults move into a long-term care setting, they must then give up their house and choose which objects to take with them from a life-time of accumulated possessions. Imagine how difficult and heart wrenching it would be to try to fit the contents of a house into a room or an apartment, especially if this is not something you really want to do. How would you decide what to take and what to leave behind? What would you do if you wanted to take a dining room set that had belonged to your grandmother, and there was no room for it in the facility? As the house and possessions are left behind, older adults usually experience what has been referred to as *de-selfing* (Goff-man, 1961). In other words, older people are not just losing a house, they are also losing a part of their sense of self. Consequently, older adults may view re-location as "an attack on self rather than an attack on property" (Krupat, 1983). This may explain the marked rise in mortality during the first year of residence in a long-term care facility that is prevalent among those who move, sometimes involuntarily, into such a setting. The move can be emotional and traumatic for many older people.

The "attack on self" varies in intensity depending on the degree to which the older adult can personalize his or her new surroundings after mov-ing into a long-term care facility. The ability to personalize often is determined by the model of care that the facility follows (see Chapter 1 for additional information on the different models of care). For example, a long-term care setting that is based on a hospital or medical model may not encourage per-sonalization. When a nursing home is envisioned more as a place to conva-lesce than as a place to reside (emphasizing *nursing* and de-emphasizing *home*), residents typically bring few possessions with them and use hospital beds and other institutional furniture provided by the facility (Figure 2.1). In addition, when residents are viewed as patients who need treatment rather than as peo-ple with individual needs, the need for personalization may not be stressed. This perception can be attributed in part to regulations. Building codes that ensure safety are designed to facilitate staff efficiency and often give little con-sideration to residents. This can affect, for example, the wall and floor finishes in residents' rooms as well as the furniture arrangements.

Similarly, a long-term care setting based on the hospitality model may provide few opportunities for personalization. In this case, a facility usually is decorated for residents, much in the same way a residential hotel would be furnished, with the intent of ensuring the residents' comfort, welcoming visi-tors, and avoiding a hospital atmosphere. Although some organizations de-liberately try to make facilities seem like hotels, resorts, or spas, others believe

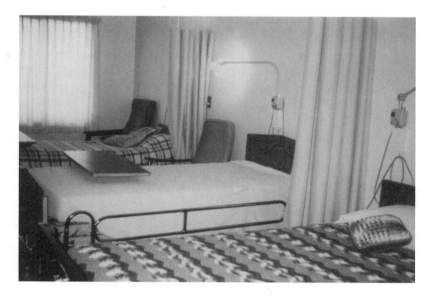

Figure 2.1.   The need for personalization may not be emphasized in a long-term care setting that uses the medical model of care.

that they are making such facilities homelike. These facilities may have bedrooms and a living room just like most homes have and may be decorated to appear homelike. Yet, these facilities are predecorated for residents and certainly would not be mistaken for a home. In other words, facilities may not realize that they are actually following the hospitality model.

The same may hold true for facilities that attempt to embrace the residential model. Based on residential housing and the treatment of older people with individual needs, the residential model stresses the need for an environment that is homelike (de-emphasizing *nursing* and emphasizing *home*). For instance, the facility may provide multiple, small dining rooms as opposed to one large dining or multipurpose room. Dining tables may be covered with tablecloths. (Synthetic fabrics usually are used because they are easier to clean and iron than are cotton or linen tablecloths.) Wood chairs with fabric seats that are similar to what is found in a house might be used. The facility may have purchased a residential china cabinet and may have put up wallpaper that coordinates with the tablecloths. These items certainly help to make a facility look nice and elegant—in some cases, nice enough to appear in a glossy interior design magazine.

Residents do not always have the chance, however, to participate in the decoration or to add their own belongings, especially to shared spaces. For instance, a facility might not want a resident to bring a chair that belonged to his or her spouse. This may be because the chair does not meet fire regulations, but it also may be because the chair does not look nice or is not contemporary. Yet that old chair may be associated with many memories and may have great sentimental value, something that cannot be achieved with a new chair provided by a facility. Consequently, the facility may be providing an environment that is generically homelike but not really reflective of the homes in which its residents lived. In other words, greater opportunities for personalization, where the self is truly taken into account, are necessary to create an environment that is more like home rather than just homelike in appearance (Calkins, 1995).

HOW DEMENTIA AFFECTS PERSONALIZATION

Imagine how difficult it must be to feel like yourself when you are losing your memory. In addition to the losses that are associated with aging and relocation, the older person with dementia also experiences a loss of cognitive functioning. Of all of the cognitive deficits associated with dementia, memory loss is most related to the self. Older adults' sense of identity is tied up with memories of a lifetime of experiences. As those memories fade, older people's sense of identity—knowing who they are as individuals—also fades. Older people can experience a profound sense of emptiness as a result, not realizing that the dementia is robbing them of their sense of self. This experience can be exacerbated by agnosia, a condition in which older people are unable to recognize or identify faces, places, objects, and events despite intact sensory abilities. Think about how frightening it would be if you could no longer remember things that you considered important—your children's names and faces or your favorite hobby.

Dementia has a different impact on memory at various stages. In the early stage, people with dementia may be able to recall most major recent events but, in general, will experience deficits in the recall of recent specific details. They usually remember many past events, although they may confuse the sequence of these events because of gaps in memory. Despite these deficits there is still continuity of the self. In the middle stage, people with dementia often cannot remember recent events and have difficulty putting thoughts into words, understanding what others are saying, and recognizing people and things. Yet their long-term memory usually remains intact, contributing to some continuity of the self. In the late stage of dementia, when recent and past memories are faint, there is some indication that emotional components of the self still remain (Coons, 1985; Feil, 1999). This suggests that some portion of the self is maintained even in late-stage dementia.

> *Myrtle always loved playing the violin. She started taking lessons at the age of 5, studied music at a college in New York, played with a philharmonic orchestra for a few years until she married, and then pursued a career as a high school music teacher after raising two children. In retirement, Myrtle continued to play the violin daily, but she began to have trouble remembering the names of former students if she ran into them in town. She also could not recall the names of past colleagues and whether she had studied with them in college or played with them in the orchestra. After Myrtle's husband died, her memory deficits worsened, and her children suggested that she move into a long-term care facility for residents with dementia. Myrtle had to leave many possessions behind when moving, but she insisted on taking her violin. As time went on, Myrtle became unsure of the weather and her current address and did not always recognize her children or grandchildren. Yet she was still able to pick up her violin and play a concerto from memory. In the late stage of dementia, when Myrtle had little knowledge of past events and could not play music any longer, she still would touch her violin lovingly from time to time. For Myrtle, there was some continuity of self throughout the progression of her dementia.*

Housing, which is an important part of older people's lives, becomes even more important to people with dementia who are losing major parts of their memory and their sense of self. This is because older people with dementia often increasingly rely on the environment for cues about how to behave. For instance, when they are brought to a room for a meal, they may know how to behave and relate to this activity only when the room looks like a dining room and dishes and food are visible. Otherwise, they may yell or attempt to leave. This stresses the importance of environmental cues that are concrete and obvious, such as china cabinets and tablecloths.

Familiar cues are important, too. After relocating to a long-term care setting, older people with dementia usually are placed in a setting that is unfamiliar in appearance and room layout. To affirm the sense of self that is intact, they need recognizable items that have some sort of emotional appeal, such as personal possessions from their past. This can stimulate the memory and ease the transition to the new setting. How else can we expect older people with dementia to adjust to a new environment? There is also a need for settings that resemble, as closely as possible, the past homes of older people. Several studies have indicated that negative effects following a move are much higher when there are marked differences between the homes that older people have to leave and the setting into which they move (Miller & Lieberman, 1965). Thus, personalization of the environment in a long-term care setting with familiar objects, familiar furniture arrangements, and residential finishes and imagery is important for residents with dementia.

> In a long-term care facility, a staff member approached Sarah, a resident, who seemed upset. "Are you lost?" the staff member asked. Sarah did not reply, so the staff member took Sarah's arm and walked with her. As they approached the door to Sarah's room, the staff member said, "See? Here's your sign, 'Flowers by Sarah.' That was the name of your store, wasn't it?" When they entered, there were many items to look at, such as photos on the wall and a distinctive pillow on the bed. Sarah sat on the bed, hugged the pillow, and stroked it from time to time. "Your sister made that pillow for your wedding," the staff member said. The staff member then pointed out several more objects. Eventually, Sarah began work on a dried flower arrangement, and the staff member felt comfortable about leaving the room.

In this case, familiar surroundings eased Sarah's anxiety. Staff also used familiar objects to help Sarah connect to the memories that remain and to remind her of who she is as an individual.

WHAT STAFF CAN DO

Staff can help increase opportunities for personalization among residents in long-term care settings in a number of ways. Some of the recommendations provided here are directed toward administrators and refer to policies that can be implemented to encourage personalization. Although these suggestions are directed at the administrative level, all staff should be involved in personalization, and their input should be considered. Other recommendations are directed more toward staff directly involved in caregiving. In this case, administration must fully support staff if these recommendations are implemented.

Many of the recommendations may require a facility to alter its thinking about what contributes to a sense of home. In particular, a facility may have to decide whether it wishes to present a tidy, elegant, formal image or whether to more actively involve residents and family members in personalizing private and shared spaces, such as dining rooms, living rooms, and courtyards, so that individual identities are represented and spaces look lived in. This is something that all levels of staff at the facility must discuss in conjunction with the model of care the facility follows, unless this is dictated by a corporate/administrative entity.

Developing Policies to Encourage Personalization

If the facility has decided to involve residents and family members actively in the personalization of the long-term care setting, then its administration should consider developing several management policies based on input from all levels of staff. These policies not only should allow residents and family members to personalize spaces but also should strongly encourage them to do so (Calkins, 1995).

The facility should consider establishing a policy regarding the personalization of bedrooms. To reflect the identity of the residents accurately, residents should be allowed to bring personal possessions, including mementos, ornaments, knickknacks, plants, and furniture. (Upholstered furniture must meet fire codes. This topic is discussed in more detail in the "What the Environment Can Do.") The facility also should allow residents and family members to hang pictures and artwork on walls and, if possible, select paint colors or wallpaper when moving in or remodeling. You may wish to provide a range of acceptable colors or patterns among which to choose.

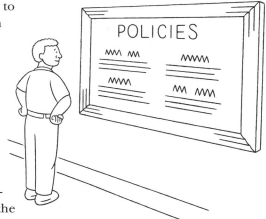

The resident's ability to personalize his or her bedroom can provide many benefits. It can help decrease the negative effects of a move to a long-term care facility, which can be a traumatic experience for older people. Because family members often experience guilt as well as sadness when placing a loved one in a long-term care setting, their active involvement may help them to view the relocation effort in a more positive way. Personalization also may reinforce the fact that family can remain a part of the older person's life. In addition to benefits for residents and family members, personalization can help staff to understand residents as individuals and understand how they lived.

Similarly, the facility should consider a policy that strongly encourages personalization in shared spaces such as living rooms or dining rooms. Although shared spaces in many facilities are decorated for residents to provide an elegant, formal, well-coordinated marketing image for visitors and family members, these types of spaces usually do not reflect the houses that older people lived in before moving to a long-term care setting. To reflect the identities of the occupants accurately, residents and family members should be permitted to contribute personal possessions such as artwork and furniture. Staff should explain to residents and family members that their contributions can encourage the use of these shared spaces and can contribute to a lived-in look. Staff also should clarify that their intention is not to cut costs by asking for residents and family members to contribute personal possessions; feelings of well-being can result when residents take a more active role in the decoration of the facility in which they live. The facility also should establish a policy for returning items to family members at a later date.

In addition, facility administration should consider a management policy that permits personalization of outdoor shared spaces such as courtyards or gardens. Facility policy should encourage residents and family members to contribute outdoor furniture, adjustable umbrellas, porch swings, lawn ornaments, bird feeders, birdhouses, wind chimes, weather vanes, and birdbaths. As with interior shared spaces, the facility should establish a policy for returning these items to family members at a later date. Management also should establish a policy that permits gardening in shared outdoor spaces. Staff might consider rewarding individual garden areas from time to time to encourage personalization. Other residents could gather and admire the gardener's work, which would help to reinforce the identity of the gardener.

Helping Residents with Personalization

This section focuses on ways that staff, particularly those who are directly involved in caregiving, can play a vital role in implementing policies that allow and encourage personalization among residents.

Gathering Information About the Resident's History

Gathering information about each resident's personal history can provide staff with a greater understanding of the residents as individuals, how they lived, and how they might wish to personalize spaces. This information-gathering process should be more extensive and intensive than that which social workers typically conduct at admission.

Ideally, staff should visit a prospective resident's current home to a get a sense of how he or she lives. In reality, most facilities cannot afford to send staff on such site visits. Consequently, staff should request information from incoming residents during admission that deals with the resident's housing history, including previous significant homes, decor preferences, and meaningful possessions. Family members can be encouraged to participate and provide photographs of the older person's home before relocation. Staff can learn about the resident's housing values (e.g., is decor important?), way of living (e.g., are neatness and organization important?), preferences (e.g., dark or light colors? contemporary or Early American furniture?), and the meanings behind certain objects (e.g., a cedar chest can be just a cedar chest to staff until they are told that the chest was given to a widow by her husband on their wedding day). The Resident's Social History and Resident's Housing History forms provided in Appendix A at the end of this volume can assist staff in gathering the necessary resident history.

In addition, social workers should consider collecting admission information a second time several weeks after the initial shock of relocation. The information likely will be more in-depth and will show residents and family members that staff do care about residents as individuals. Admission is a stressful time for both residents and family members, especially because a crisis may have prompted the need for an older person to move to a facility.

For residents already living in long-term care settings, staff can gather information by meeting with each resident and his or her family members and asking them about the resident's social, family, and housing history. In the process, staff can emphasize the importance of personalization and its therapeutic benefits for people with memory loss. To document the information that is gathered from these sessions, family members can be encouraged to label photographs or to assemble an annotated poster or collage highlighting the resident's life, which can be placed in his or her bedroom. Large print and color contrast should be used for captions. Text should be simple for residents with dementia. Photographs, posters, or collages not only will remind staff of each resident's history but also will help staff view residents as people in the context of a whole life (Figure 2.2).

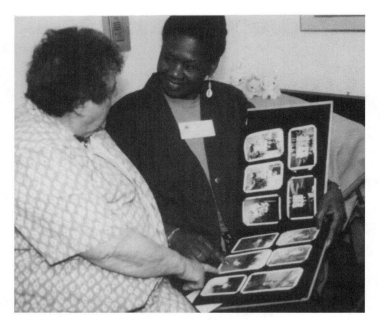

Figure 2.2.   Viewing a photo album can give staff a sense of the resident as a person in the context of his or her life and remind them of the resident's history.

Reminiscing

Reminiscing is often an enjoyable activity for individuals with dementia, especially because their long-term memory remains intact for a much longer period of time. With a greater understanding of residents as individuals, staff can use residents' personal mementos, knickknacks, or reminiscing art provided by the facility to prompt conversations among residents and staff. These can help residents remember important people and events in their lives and retain information about themselves in the process. (See "Where to Find Products" for sources of reminiscing art.)

In addition, staff can redirect residents who may be upset or are being disruptive by showing them familiar items that are used to personalize spaces. When staff have an understanding of residents as individuals, they will know which personal possessions are most likely to please residents, interest them, and make them happy. They also will be able to remind residents why certain possessions are important. For example, a staff member may be able to point out a quilt that a family member made. Staff should be aware, however, that it is sometimes difficult to know or predict whether an object will evoke positive or negative memories for residents with dementia. For instance, a war medal may evoke proud feelings for one resident who served his country during World War II, whereas it may remind another resident of being a prisoner of war. It is best when staff have several items among which to choose.

Staff must realize that reminiscing is an ongoing process, and they may have to be creative in coming up with different solutions to engage residents in it. For example, even when staff are aware of a resident's likes and dislikes because they know the resident well, the resident may be having a bad day, and what worked before may not work now. The resident's needs also may change as the dementia progresses. Staff may have to think about engaging residents in reminiscing and personalization that relates to the parts of the residents' past lives that they believe they are living in now. Having mementos from different periods of a resident's life can help. This ongoing process is an important part of a caregiver's job, and can ensure a better quality of life for residents in the process. Administration should reinforce this and let staff know that this type of caregiving does make a difference.

Decorating

In addition, staff can involve residents actively in personalization as an activity. For example, residents' artwork can be displayed in hallways. Residents who are more cognitively intact and who have been interested in art could help decide where to hang the work and how to arrange it on the walls. Similarly, some residents may be interested in actually hanging the artwork. This may give residents who were used to handling tools such as a hammer a chance to engage in a familiar activity. However, staff should be certain that these residents are calm rather than agitated, because a hammer is a potentially hazardous tool.

WHAT THE ENVIRONMENT CAN DO

This section offers ideas for increasing opportunities for personalization in long-term care settings through their physical features. Both the insides and outsides of buildings are taken into account. The more private areas of the facility are discussed first by examining residents' bedrooms, private bathrooms, and bedroom entries. Next, personalization of residents' bedrooms from the outside is examined by addressing the exterior windows. Finally, indoor and outdoor shared spaces in the facility, including living rooms, dining rooms, lobbies, and outdoor courtyards and garden areas, are reviewed.

Residents' Bedrooms

In some long-term care facilities, individual bedrooms may be furnished and decorated for residents before they move into the facility. Walls may be papered and coordinated with curtains, bedspreads, and carpeting using fashionable colors. Furniture that looks residential also may be provided. As described in Chapter 1, using residential decor, finishes, and lighting and minimizing the visibility of institutional features such as linen carts and alarms can contribute to a homelike appearance. Although this is important, bedrooms that are picture perfect do not truly reflect the identity of the occupants and certainly are not mistaken by residents for home. Many older adults have never lived in such color-coordinated, perfect environments (Calkins, 1995).

Just as in a house, the bedroom is the most personal area of a long-term care setting. It should be a place where older people can arrange furniture and select decorations that they like. Most important, the bedroom should be comfortable and feel like the resident's own. This can be accomplished in many ways—ranging from the display of meaningful objects and the arrangement of furniture to the selection of paint colors.

Create Places for Ornaments and Knickknacks

Staff can encourage residents to bring from home personal mementos, ornaments, knickknacks, and framed photographs, especially those to which they have a strong personal attachment. As discussed earlier, these objects are extremely important as connections to the individual's historical past. They can evoke memories and can be used to express and preserve residents' sense of self. Some examples might include a china doll collection, a set of crystal wine glasses that belonged to a close relative, or a plaque documenting an older person's military service during a war.

The facility should provide places to accommodate the display of these meaningful objects. Wide window ledges and flat furniture tops are examples. Built-in shelves would be ideal but are difficult to implement in existing buildings. Constructing shelves or a cabinet in a corner of the bedroom might be more feasible, especially because corners are underused. Shelves that can be protected by glass doors that open and close may help to prevent residents from "borrowing" personal items from other people. High shelves that keep more precious, breakable items visible but less accessible might also serve this function (Figure 2.3). Some possessions, however, should be placed at a height so that residents can see and handle the items without being tempted

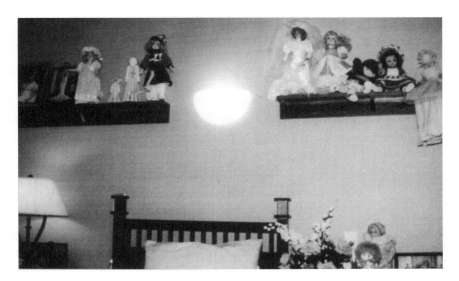

Figure 2.3.   A resident's doll collection can be displayed on shelves that are out of residents' reach for protection.

to climb on furniture. In all cases, lighting levels should be bright enough so that residents can see these items. (See "Where to Find Products" for sources of good-quality lighting.)

Hang Pictures and Artwork

The facility should encourage the display of pictures or other wall hangings. These might include pieces of art collected over the years, blankets or rugs acquired from travel to other countries, or even pictures made by children or grandchildren. Pictures and wall hangings should be attached firmly to walls so that residents will not be able to remove them. Should holes in the wall be a concern, a picture rail or shelf can be added around the perimeter of the wall for hanging pictures. (Instructions for creating a picture shelf and hanging rod are provided in Appendix B. Sources of wall hanging systems are provided in "Where to Find Products.") Residents, family, or both should have the option of deciding on the placement of wall hangings. (Create your own economical hanging system by fastening a strip of wood or molding to the wall and using wires and screws fastened to the top to hang artwork [see Appendix B]. Wood strips can be painted or covered with wall covering borders for a finished look.)

Use Personal Furniture and Familiar Arrangements

If personal furniture is sturdy and in good condition, then residents and family should be encouraged to bring a few pieces to the facility. As with wall hangings, residents should have the option of deciding on the placement of furniture. Some may want to replicate the furniture layout of their previous home as much as possible. Replication helps the environment seem more familiar and may help confused residents feel less disoriented. It also prevents residents with low vision from bumping into furnishings. Replication might be more difficult, however, when the resident shares a room with another person.

Residents should be encouraged to bring from home sufficient numbers of table and floor lamps that they can turn on and off depending on the desired light level, in addition to the typical chair and dresser. In many cases, overhead fluorescent lighting is already provided. This type of lighting does provide ambient light but in general is not homelike. It should be supplemented with table or floor lamps, which are more homelike and provide lighting to help residents with specific tasks when placed next to a chair or a bed. Some of these lamps can be attached to tables to make them sturdier.

Add Natural Plants

Residents should be encouraged to bring plants from home, especially if gardening was a favorite activity. Plants can serve as a direct connection to nature and can provide an opportunity for older people to care for something. Living things can be therapeutic. The Eden Alternative program (Thomas, 1996) stresses that plants should be incorporated within the daily life of a facility to promote growth among residents. In addition, the colors, textures, and fragrances of plants can brighten a room. Although natural plants are more desirable than silk plants, staff must remember that residents with middle- and late-stage dementia often put things in their mouths, including flowers and plants. Thus, staff should make sure that all natural plants brought from previous homes are nontoxic (Brawley, 1997). (See Appendix C for a list of toxic plants.) With the assistance of family members or staff, residents can place plants on wide window ledges, flat furniture tops, and plant stands or hang plants from ceilings.

Offer a Variety of Finishes

Although bringing mementos and furniture from a previous home are some of the most common forms of personalization and are undoubtedly important, personalization should not be limited to personal furniture and knickknacks. Yet, many facilities provide bedrooms with identical colors and identical wall, ceiling, and floor finishes that inhibit additional personalization. Often, these items are neutral in color as if to stress the nonidentity of the occupants.

If possible, the facility should develop three or four different color schemes for wall finishes from which residents can choose. Rooms need to be painted periodically and usually are painted before a new resident takes occupancy. Because this is the resident's only personal space, it is important that his or her color preferences are taken into account. This can be accomplished by talking with residents and family members and providing them with 8½-inch by 11-inch samples of the available wall finishes (easier to see than small paint chips). If residents, particularly those with dementia, do not understand or are not able to articulate color preferences, then they can be provided with different-colored objects (e.g., fabric swatches) and observed to determine which colors they pick up and handle most often. In general, it is advantageous if adjacent resident bedrooms are painted different colors so that residents do not become confused.

When assembling different color schemes from which residents can choose, you might want to determine how warm or cool the color of the bedrooms feel. Often, this feeling depends on the orientation of the rooms to the position of the sun and wind and on the heating and cooling systems. Although little research has been conducted on the psychological effects of color on older people with dementia, there is some indication that bright, warm colors such as reds, oranges, and peaches make rooms that are habitually cool in actual temperature seem warmer. These colors also help to make people look healthier and less sallow than colors on the cooler end of the spectrum. When rooms already are warm, cooler colors such as blues and greens may be more appropriate.

Whatever paint colors are selected, the use of an eggshell paint finish is recommended. This finish decreases the amount of reflected glare that is typical with a glossy finish. A wall painted with eggshell paint is also easier to clean than a flat paint finish. In addition, color contrast between walls and floors is important (see Volume 2 for details). In general, dark colors absorb light and make it more difficult for residents with vision problems to see well. Finally, consider colors that were popular among residents in their previous homes. One survey of older adults in long-term care facilities in central Ohio (Zavotka & Teaford, 1998) revealed that brown, yellow, blue, and green were the colors used most often in older adults' homes. Using these colors, at least in the surveyed Ohio facilities, could be a familiar cue for residents; however, they might not be regionally appropriate in Miami or Tucson.

Paint colors also can be used in conjunction with a variety of wallpaper and border patterns. These do not have to be extremely well coordinated because most residents did not have homes that were like model homes. At the same time, a variety of colors can relieve monotony, provide some visual stimulation, and emphasize the uniqueness of each resident's bedroom. Where paint colors are fixed, borders are an inexpensive addition that can help to enhance identity.

Let Residents Choose Their Own Fabrics

Fire regulation codes, which vary from state to state and by facility type, may stipulate that bedspreads and drapery fabrics be fire rated. If this is the case, then the facility should consider providing several different bedspreads and window curtains from which residents and families can choose. These options can be coordinated with the wall and ceiling color scheme that is selected by residents. Facilities should choose patterns carefully. Certain wavy, undulating patterns may appear to move and cause residents with dementia to experience unsteadiness. Some residents also may become dizzy or disoriented by large geometric patterns. In general, it is advantageous to choose small patterns and to test these out in one area first to see how residents react. Unfortunately, research is sparse in this area, and there is no single correct solution. In some cases, residents and family members may be able to bring bedspreads or quilts and curtains from home if they can be made flame retardant by a professional fabric finisher.

Private Bathrooms

Offer a Variety of Finishes

As with finishes in residents' bedrooms, the finishes in individual bathrooms should be residential in nature. For instance, residents should have the opportunity to select from a variety of wall color schemes. It is important to select colors for the floor and walls that will contrast with the toilet. (Volume 2, Chapter 4 covers the necessity for this contrast in more detail.) Once again, paint colors can be used in conjunction with a variety of wallpaper and border patterns. If the facility cannot repaint or re-paper bathrooms, adding borders and decorative towels that are selected by residents can help to enhance identity.

Add Personal Items

Residents can add personal items to private bathrooms as well. A shelf over the sink could be provided for old perfume and lotion bottles, hairbrushes, and shampoos. Residents who were avid gardeners also could add plants that do well in moist environments. (A grow light may be necessary in bathrooms without windows.) These suggestions may not be appropriate in all cases because of space constraints or the possibility of residents ingesting items or putting them in the toilet. At the very least, residents should be encouraged to display art on bathroom walls and to hang curtains around windows and tubs if they are present. In addition, residents can select room fresheners or aromatherapy oils to make bathrooms smell pleasant (see "Where to Find Products" for sources of aromatherapy products).

Bedroom Entryways

Have you ever had difficulty finding your room in a hotel? All of the hallways and doors looked the same, and you may have found yourself relying on signs and room numbers. In a similar way, having many resident bedroom doors opening onto hallways in a long-term care facility can detract from the residents' ability to identify their rooms as uniquely theirs. As a result, it may be necessary to use some sort of personalization to differentiate one room from another. Such personalization of the entry can enhance residents' sense of self and help them lay claim to their bedrooms. The bedroom door is usually the best place to mark a room as belonging to a particular resident because this is where a transition occurs from shared space to personal space in a facility. In addition, personalization can help confused residents identify their bedrooms (Volume 2, Chapter 2 addresses this issue in detail). Personalizing the bedroom entry can be accomplished by decorating front doors and adding display cases.

Decorate Front Doors

The bedroom entry can be made more personal if it is decorated just as a front door to a single-family house would be decorated. Wreaths, welcome signs, and nameplates can be added to the door itself, as can more personal items such as a small piece of needlepoint made by the resident or a collage of photos of the resident, family members, or a favorite pet. Staff should make sure that these items are placed in an area and at a height at which a resident is most likely to see them. For example, if a resident uses a wheelchair or is stooped over when walking, then the display item should be placed at that resident's eye level. In facilities where bedroom doors are recessed, residents can add a doormat and a shelf or small piece of furniture for plants or other small knickknacks. Residents and their families must understand, however, that objects on a shelf or a piece of furniture could be "borrowed" by other residents.

Add Display Cases

Display cases can take the form of shadow boxes, curio cabinets, or display cabinets. Shadow boxes, in which the outside glass is approximately 2 inches away from the back of the frame, can hold small mementos such as war medals or figurines. Curio cabinets can be open cabinets with multiple shelves or closed cabinets with glass doors. Both shadow boxes and curio cabinets usually are applied to a wall, but they should not jut out into the hallway more than 4 inches. They should have glare-free glass to enhance the visibility of objects. Display cabinets usually are larger and deeper and can hold larger items such as religious statues or trophies (Figure 2.4). These cabinets usually are recessed (built into the wall so that they do not project out into the hallway more than 4 inches), but this placement can be restricted by wall construction, building codes, and costs. The facility should check building codes before implementing such a modification. In all cases, lighting should be adequate for residents to see the display items. (See "Where to Find Products" for sources for shadow boxes. You can also check with local home furnishings stores for display cases.)

Exterior Window Treatments

When you approach your own house after a day's work, you can probably identify your bedroom or your child's bedroom by the different sizes of exterior windows or the decorations around them. In a long-term care facility, this can be a bit more difficult. Often, residents' rooms are represented on the outside of the building by many identical windows. This arrangement can detract from the residents' identity. To encourage individual identity of residents' rooms from the outside, staff can encourage personalization even when the window design itself is unchangeable. Residents or family members can add a personal touch to windows with curtains or drapes, hanging plants, and suncatchers as well as by placing ornaments or plants on windowsills that are

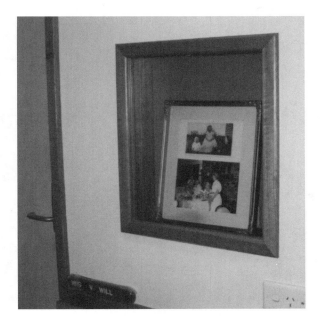

Figure 2.4. A display cabinet containing a resident's personal photographs can be used to personalize the entrance to the resident's bedroom.

visible from the outside. In addition, the facility can add window boxes for flowers and plants, especially if they can be tended from inside the unit. These suggestions can help to reduce the monotony associated with expansive building exteriors without destroying the building's overall appearance.

Interior Shared Spaces

Typically, facilities are decorated and furnished for residents before they move into a long-term care setting. This is even more likely to happen in shared spaces of the facility, such as the dining area or lobby. Here, formal furniture, silk plants, and well-coordinated accessories may be used to present a good public relations/marketing image for family members and visitors. In addition, day rooms and lounges may be referred to as living rooms or family rooms, and lobbies may be called foyers. Sometimes, residential decor and terminology can contribute to a homelike appearance, especially when the visibility of institutional features such as linen carts, alarms, and control panels also is minimized. However, long-term care facilities that are decorated with elegant and well-coordinated fabrics and finishes are probably not like

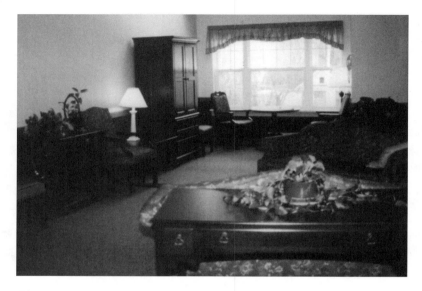

Figure 2.5. Well-coordinated, elegant interior spaces are probably not like the houses that residents lived in before relocating to a long-term care facility.

the houses the residents lived in before relocating. These types of facilities would not be mistaken for home (see Figure 2.5).

Personalization of the public areas of a long-term care setting may help to make a facility more like home by reflecting the identities of the individual occupants. Opportunities for personalization also may encourage the use of these shared spaces. After all, residents do not live just in their bedrooms. They usually use a public dining room every day and should use other shared spaces as well.

Decorate with Residents' Possessions

Personalization of shared spaces can be accomplished by encouraging residents and family members to bring possessions with them from their previous homes for the public areas of the facility. For example, a china cabinet or a breakfront in the dining room and a grandfather clock in the foyer are appropriate choices. Bookcases, wall units, or curio cabinets also could be used to display residents' memorabilia. Staff might consider featuring a different resident's memorabilia each month in display cases as a kind of rotating exhibition. Staff could hang artwork on walls as well, especially in corridors. This can enhance an individual's sense of identity and help to develop a sense of community in the process. Furthermore, such displays add variety and interest to each room—a true reflection of a home—and can aid confused residents with orientation.

Combine Residents' Possessions with Residential-Style Purchases

Reflecting many identities can be challenging in a group living arrangement. Issues of territoriality may arise with furniture, such as a favorite chair, or with particular possessions. In addition, residents and family members may not feel comfortable placing furnishings or objects of even modest economic or sentimental value in a public place. In this case, the facility may have to purchase some items to decorate shared spaces.

If the facility is considering buying new furniture, a number of manufacturers make commercial-grade, highly durable furniture that looks residential. It is a good idea to purchase furniture that is somewhat similar to the furniture that residents would bring into the facility. Because many people purchase their furniture a piece or a room at a time, furnishings need not match exactly in terms of the wood type, wood color, or fabric color and pattern. In other words, do not overdecorate. An eclectic look and rooms with many different but coordinated pieces of furniture are much more like the homes with which the residents have identified over a lifetime. Furthermore, this can result in a less formal and cozier look. As with a family home, residents should feel as if they can put their feet on the furniture if they would like.

Tub Room

On occasion, every resident must use the tub room. Private bathrooms may not include a tub or shower area, and some residents may need assistance with bathing. Personalization may help to decrease agitation in residents who are combative during bathing and help to create a more homelike room in the process. Staff should consider talking with families of residents who are particularly challenging to bathe to determine whether any particular features in a bathroom might help to make a difference. For example, residents may wish to bring along their own decorative towel or contribute a piece of bathroom art. If there is space in the tub room, then a grooming area with a vanity, seat, and mirror can add residential character. Creating a grooming area might be as simple as providing a table with a skirt. Shampoos, soaps, and lotions can be placed in this area. Be sure the lighting is sufficient. This is one area where incandescent bulbs, which generally reflect warm and healthful-looking skin tones, should be considered.

Outdoor Shared Spaces

As with interior shared spaces, outdoor spaces also should reflect the identities of the individual occupants to increase comfort and familiarity and to encourage the use of these areas as an extension of the indoor environment. Residents and family members should be encouraged to bring possessions with them from their previous homes for the outdoor public areas of the facility. For example, outdoor furniture such as picnic tables, adjustable umbrellas, and porch swings as well as lawn ornaments, bird feeders, birdhouses, birdbaths, wind chimes, and weather vanes are appropriate choices.

Issues of territoriality may arise, however, with possessions and certain pieces of furniture. For instance, residents who were used to sitting on a porch swing with family members in the context of their previous house may have difficulty sharing the same porch swing with a stranger in the long-term care facility. In addition, residents and family members may not feel comfortable placing furnishings or objects of even modest economic or sentimental value in a public place. In this case, the facility may purchase outdoor furniture to supplement the possessions from previous homes that are donated by residents (see "Where to Find Products" for sources). Any outdoor furniture that is purchased should be residential in style and should be made of nonreflective materials to minimize glare.

Other ways to create opportunities for personalization include individual gardening areas. High-functioning residents should be encouraged to transplant some of the plantings from the gardens in their previous homes to their individual gardening areas in the long-term care setting. Along with family members, residents can continue to tend and add to these areas. This activity provides an opportunity for reminiscence as well as support for interaction between residents and families. If residents cannot bring plants with them, then ask about their favorite plants and flowers and incorporate some of these in the garden (Zeisel & Tyson, 1999).

Garden areas should include planter beds that are placed at varying heights or that gradually slope and are accessible at different heights. This allows each gardener, including those who use wheelchairs, to select an appropriate working area. Raised planters are also easier to view without stooping (see "Where to Find Products" for sources for gardening products). In addition, staff might consider rewarding individual garden areas from time to time to encourage personalization. Other residents could gather to admire the gardener's work, which would help to reinforce the identity of the gardener. Easily accessible storage areas for gardening tools, supplied by either the residents or their family members and checked by the facility to ensure safety, should be provided. Access to nearby water and opportunities for seating, preferably in both sun and shade, also is necessary.

Although low-functioning residents may not be able to participate actively in such gardening activities, they can be brought outside to look at the gardens and to enjoy the warmth of the sun and the familiar aromas. Incorporating features that will attract birds—particularly songbirds in the area—also provides positive stimulation for residents with more severe impairment.

WHERE TO FIND PRODUCTS

Interactive and Reminiscing Art

3D Interactive Art by Mardel DeBuhr Sanzotta
84 Fruitland Avenue
Painesville, OH 44077
(216) 357-7122
Tactile artwork with some interactive items

Artline
W227 North 937 Westmound Drive
Waukesha, WI 53186
(800) 795-9596
www.artline.com
Interactive and memory-based artwork

DesignXpertise Studio
1700 Mary Street
Pittsburgh, PA 15203
(412) 431-5733
www.designxpertise.com
Memory quilts and memory boxes by artist Karen Scofield

Lighting

Architectural Lighting Systems
30 Sherwood Drive
Taunton, MA 02780
(508) 823-8277
Cove lighting

Holophane Co.
214 Oakwood Avenue
Newark, OH 43055
(740) 345-9631
Baffles for fluorescent lights

Microsun, Inc.
(800) 657-0077
www.microsun.com
Floor and table lamps that use combination incandescent and metal halide lamps to provide high-efficiency, high-level lighting

Adjustable Fixture Co.
3726 North Booth Street
Milwaukee, WI 53212
(800) 558-2628
www.adjustablefixture.com
Table and floor lamps

SPI Lighting Inc.
10400 North Enterprise Drive
Mequon, WI 53092
(414) 242-1420
www.spilighting.com
Wall sconces that meet the Americans with Disabilities Act of 1990 (PL 101-336) 4-inch clearance standard and come with a variety of lighting options

Aromatherapy

Gaiam
(formerly Selfcare)
360 Interlocken Boulevard, Suite 300
Broomfield, CO 80021-3440
(877) 989-6321
www.gaiam.com

Wall Hanging Systems that Avoid Making Holes in a Wall

Conwed Designscape
800 Gustafson Road
Ladysmith, WI 54848
(800) 932-2383
www.conweddesignscape.com
Tack hole wall coverings

Exposures, Inc.
Post Office Box 3615
Oshkosh, WI 54903-3615
(800) 222-4947
www.exposuresonline.com
Picture hanging rods and display ledges

JM Lynne Co., Inc.
59 Gilpin Avenue
Post Office Box 1010
Smithtown, NY 11787
(800) 645-5044
www.jmlynne.com
Velcro-compatible wall coverings

Shadow Boxes

Exposures, Inc.
Post Office Box 3615
Oshkosh, WI 54903-3615
(800) 222-4947
www.exposuresonline.com
A catalog of items for the storage and display of photographs and mementos

Outdoor Furniture

Fincastle County Chairworks
2821 South English Station Road
Louisville, KY 40299
(502) 267-1888
Resin furniture that looks like wood but will not deteriorate

Leisure Woods
Post Office Box 177
Genoa, IL 60135
(800) 422-9326

Marin Deck Chair
230 Arroyo Road
Lagunitas, CA 94938-0294
(415) 488-4477
www.sunorshade.com
Chaise de Soleil outdoor glider

WhisperGLIDE
10051 Kerry Court
Hugo, MN 55038
(800) 944-7737
www.whisperglide.com
WhisperGLIDE outdoor glider swing

Gardening

StandUp Gardens, Ltd.
34 Patterson Lane
Portsmouth, NH 03801
(800) TO-STAND
www.standupgardens.com
A portable gardening area that can be used indoors or out, does not require residents to stoop, and provides a gardening experience for residents with various capabilities

◆ ◆ ◆

A summary sheet follows, which condenses the chapter text into a quick overview. The authors have also provided an area for you to make your own notes about your own staff and facility. Managerial staff may wish to use the summary sheets as handouts to accompany direct care staff training, or to post them by the time clock or nurses' station or include them in staff's pay envelopes.

PERSONALIZATION SUMMARY SHEET

1. Personalization is an expression of self.
2. Personal memorabilia tell others what a person has done, what is important, and what he or she likes or dislikes.
3. Personalization makes up a resident's life story, and provides a connection to his or her past.
4. Using personal objects in residents' rooms helps make rooms or spaces that are similar more distinct and different from one another, helps mark a territory as a resident's own, and helps define how a space should be used.

What Staff Can Do

1. Help develop and support policies that promote personalization in bedrooms, shared spaces, and outdoor spaces.
2. Use personal items in reminiscing with residents.
3. Try to arrange furniture as close as possible to the way it was arranged at the resident's previous home.

What the Environment Can Do

1. Provide places to put ornaments and knickknacks (shelves, wide window sills, systems to hang pictures).
2. Provide options in resident room decor (e.g., wall color, curtains, bedspreads, furniture styles).
3. Provide spaces to personalize, and decorate entryways to bedrooms.
4. Provide personal garden area or a large planter for each resident.

YOUR NOTES

3
Roles and Activities

When Susan woke up this morning, she took a shower, got dressed, and made her bed. She prepared breakfast for her children and packed their lunches before they left for school. She managed to catch a few minutes of the morning news on television and then commuted to her job as an aide in a nursing facility. After a busy day running around and caring for residents, she stopped at the garden center to buy some flowers, hoping that she might get to do a little gardening that evening. She would have liked to spend more time

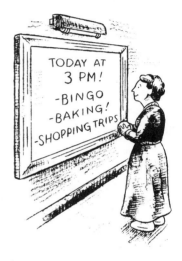

shopping, but she had to pick up her daughter from the child care center and her son from baseball practice at school. When she arrived home and got out of her car, her neighbor spotted her from his porch and walked over to chat for a few minutes. Susan gave her house keys to her son so that her children could go inside the house. A few minutes later, Susan's son told her that her brother was on the telephone. Susan then spent a good half hour talking to her brother so that they could plan their father's 75th birthday party.

Like Susan, you probably did many things today. A day in your life was probably just as full with activities, routines, and interactions related to many different areas of your life. When Susan made her bed and prepared breakfast for her family, for example, she participated in domestic activities or routines related to self-care and the maintenance of her home. Taking care of residents in the nursing facility was part of Susan's paid, productive work.

When Susan chatted with her neighbor and planned a birthday party for her father, she took part in leisure or social interests.

As with Susan, your social roles are derived from activities and routines from different parts of your life. Susan's role as a parent, for instance, was evident when she prepared breakfast for her children and picked her son up from baseball practice. Her roles as a sibling and an adult child were reinforced as she planned a birthday party for her father with her brother. She was also a neighbor, a friend, and an employee. The activities from different parts of your life as well as the roles you hold are important. In combination, they provide you with a definition of self—letting you and others know who you are. They are also basic components of psychological and social well-being.

DEFINITION OF SELF

For many of us, our homes and all of their contents—family treasures, personal possessions, decor, and furniture—are an important part of who we are as individuals. These items are a part of our lives and are ways to represent the self to others (see also Chapter 2 in this volume). However, if you have just moved and have not had a chance to unpack, then others might have some trouble trying to gain insight into the type of person you are—your values, tastes, and identity. Of course, *you* still know who you are. You might feel a bit unsettled in your new place, but you are still an employee, a parent, a sibling, or the captain of a bowling team. You are still able to participate in many activities, such as bike riding, baking, or talking on the telephone with friends with whom you have been involved for some time. In other words, the self is not represented just by personal possessions—it is also defined by roles and activities.

Some roles, such as sibling or child, are assigned to people. Others are achieved through skills and effort. Being an employee, the president of the PTA, or the coach of a soccer team are roles that people can choose and work toward. Sometimes, however, people's life experiences can influence the roles that they accept and reject. Someone who lost a parent to cancer when he or she was a child, for example, might have decided to become a nurse or a social worker as an adult. Other times, people's backgrounds can restrict their choice of roles. Those who cannot afford to go to college might have fewer job choices. Others who do not have to worry about their income might be able to devote more time to work as volunteers. In addition, some people may feel that they must assume certain roles. Many women are expected to be the caregivers in their families because women are usually associated with this role. Although societal expectations are changing as more women join the workforce, and certain roles are being shared equally between both genders, many roles were divided by gender for earlier generations.

Participating in activities that are related to work, the family, and home, as well as other social relationships and leisure interests, helps to reinforce these roles. Filling out a time sheet at work is necessary as an employee; holding a soccer practice in preparation for a game is part of being a coach; helping children with their homework is something that a parent does; and taking an aging parent grocery shopping is what most people feel they should do as loving adult children. Were you unable to participate in these types of activities, you would probably experience role loss. For instance, if you were to get a divorce and your former spouse and children moved away, then your role and identity as a parent would certainly change. Thus, activities—work, domestic, and leisure—as well as their associated roles, accumulated over a lifetime, help to provide us with a definition of self or a sense of identity.

WELL-BEING

If you were to change jobs and move to another state, then you would experience many role and activity changes. You might not live near your parents, siblings, or friends, which would have an impact on your roles as an adult child, brother or sister, and friend. You might have to get used to a new home and might have to invent new ways for continuing the domestic activities you used to do in your former home. For example, the kitchen in your new apartment might be small, making it difficult for you to bake. You also might have to go to the movies alone or simply sit home and watch television if you do not know anyone living in your new neighborhood. All in all, you might not be happy while you adjust to these changes. That is because our roles and activities not only provide us with a definition of self but also help to provide us with a sense of self-worth.

People's sense of self-worth is often based on the roles that they accept and reject throughout their lifetimes. When we are able to choose roles and are happy with the choices that we have made, we usually feel good about ourselves. When these roles are related to meaningful relationships and inclusion within supportive groups, we also feel good about ourselves. Participating in activities that reinforce these roles is important. Activities of some kind are necessary to satisfy our need to stay busy and useful. In fact, people create activity when none exists. For example, some people need to putter around the house while catching a few glimpses of what is on television, sorting through the mail, and cleaning up a little here and there, whereas others may be content to just sit and watch television. When we participate in activities that also make us feel that we have a purpose and are worthwhile, productive, contributing members of society, self-esteem is enhanced and feelings of well-being result. This is true with respect to many aspects of life, including domestic (e.g., cooking, raking leaves, activities of daily living), work (e.g., paid jobs, volunteering), and leisure (e.g., reading, swimming) activities.

Within the domestic environment, for example, people often enjoy taking care of their homes and families. Decorating the living room, gardening in the front yard, and cooking dinner for the children can provide a sense of accomplishment or pride. The home also can be the center of loving relationships with family that can contribute to feelings of warm interaction and belonging. With respect to the paid work environment, American society places great emphasis on productivity. For some people, work is just a job that involves activities one must do to earn a paycheck. For other people, work is a career that involves activities that they find personally satisfying (Kimmel, 1990). In all cases, work and productivity are linked to feelings of self-sufficiency and survival. They also are linked to our self-concept and status. Others often judge us by what work we do or what position we hold. In American culture, one of the first things people ask on meeting someone new is, "What do you do?" People may form friendships in that context and develop a sense of belonging in the process (Proffitt, 1993).

Leisure activities usually are chosen freely and typically are not related to one's work (Kimmel, 1990). Leisure may include being active (e.g., bike riding) or being quiet and passive (e.g., watching a movie). It can be something that we pursue alone (e.g., reading) or in a group (e.g., meeting friends for dinner at a restaurant). It can also be structured (e.g., card game) or unstructured (e.g., painting) and exciting or routine. In all cases, we gain satisfaction from the activity itself, the socialization involved, the opportunities for introspection and relaxation, or the learning that can take place. In addition, some people may participate in leisure activities that provide external benefits such as prestige or status. Going to the opera or an exclusive cocktail party may be particularly enjoyable to some because they like to be seen.

HOW ROLES AND ACTIVITIES CHANGE WITH AGE AND RELOCATION

Participation in work-related, domestic, and leisure activities and the roles that are derived from these activities remains important throughout life. With aging, however, older adults often experience many significant losses, such as the death of loved ones, retirement, and physical changes, that can reduce the quality and quantity of activities in which older people can engage. Such losses can lead to role loss as well, and to the related erosion of identity and self-worth. At the same time, life-cycle changes can result in older people taking on new roles and participating in new activities, such as grandparenting—taking grandchildren to the movies or watching them play soccer—that they might not have been involved in before. In addition, many older people can experience role confusion (Emlet, Crabtree, Condon, & Treml, 1996). Each of these changes is described in more detail in the following text.

Loss of Roles and Activities

Shari noticed that the number of people in her father's life continuously shrank as he aged. Her father lost his parents when he was in his early 40s. Shari moved out after getting married. Even though she lives only a couple of hours away, she is busy with her own family and job. Her brother Eric moved out when he took a job in another state. He can afford to fly home only two or three times a year. When her father reached his 60s, he retired from work and did not stay in touch with co-workers he had seen every day for years. Several years later, he lost a brother, and he has also heard of or read about former co-workers and friends who have passed away. In his 70s, he saw a couple of close neighbors moved in with their children, moved to a warmer climate, or exchanged their houses for apartments in another neighborhood. Eventually, Shari's mother died and her father had to adjust to being a widower.

Shari's father must cope with the loss of many roles. As a result of the death of loved ones, he lost the roles of adult child, sibling, spouse, and friend. When his close neighbors moved away, he also lost his role as a member of their community. Although he has maintained his role as a parent, he has had to deal with a reduction in this role because of the geographical distance that separates him from his children. In addition, retirement from work resulted in the loss of his roles as employee and co-worker.

The loss of all of these roles has an impact on activities. When Shari's father became a widower, for example, he lost the companionship of his wife and no longer has someone to share in domestic and leisure activities. As a widower, he may not be able to fit in with his remaining friends who are still part of a couple, and may experience reduced opportunities for leisure activities as a result. In addition, physical changes such as losses in sensory capacity, a reduced energy level, and the onset of chronic diseases that have an impact on mobility may have reduced Shari's father's ability and desire to participate in all kinds of activities. For instance, because he is hard of hearing, it is difficult for him to carry on a conversation with friends in a social situation. He often finds it impossible to discriminate between background noise and the voice of the person with whom he is talking. Shari's father also may be concerned about incontinence and the availability of public restrooms, places to rest while walking, or getting lost if he leaves his home to go to church or do grocery shopping.

Such losses of roles and activities can strip older people of their identity and sense of purpose. Aside from the loss in self-esteem older people can experience by not contributing to society or taking part in social interactions, plain inactivity also can have physical consequences for older people "in terms of muscles wasting, loss of joint range, and cardiopulmonary and circulatory problems" (Zgola, 1990, p. 150).

New Roles and Activities

Despite the losses in roles and activities that are typical for most older people, they also may gain some new roles and activities as they age. The birth of grandchildren resulted in a new role for Shari's father as described previously. However, as in this case, some older adults do not live in the same city or state as their grandchildren. They may not get to participate in grandparenting as they would like, but they are still grandparents. Conversely, many older adults do live in the same town as their grandchildren and help to raise them because of the need for dual incomes in many families and the desire of both women and men to have careers.

The search for new roles often follows the loss of other roles. Following retirement, for instance, many men find that they have a great deal of time on their hands. Some may seem lost and find that they have little to do because they did not develop hobbies or interests outside their work environment. They may stay at home with their wives and try to share in domestic activities such as cooking. For example, to feel some sense of purpose and usefulness, a retired man may reorganize the kitchen cabinets, infringing on his wife's territory and driving her absolutely crazy in the process. In contrast, others may search for new roles outside the home. They may start actively volunteering in a local hospital, become more involved in their church, or even get a part-time job. They may also take up golf or travel.

Role Confusion

Role confusion can occur with aging. In the preceding example, Shari's father retained the role of father, but the importance of this role changed once his children moved away. His place in the family structure is different as a result. He was accustomed to offering guidance or demanding that his children follow his advice or rules. As adults, however, his children may not do so. Shari's father may find this troubling and feel that some meaning in his life has been lost.

Such role confusion can occur with retirement as well. Shari's father may have been used to being the breadwinner in the family and working long hours with little time for domestic or leisure activities. Her mother took care of the house and the children. After retiring, her father may not have known what to do with himself or how to fit within the family structure, so he may have tried to take over his wife's role and responsibility for the house.

Relocation

Garrett is forced to stay in a hotel room for an entire week for a business trip. After three nights of eating in the hotel restaurant, he relishes the thought of a home-cooked meal. Unfortunately, he must wait until he gets home because the hotel room is not equipped with a kitchen. At the very least, he wishes that he could have a glass of milk before going to bed. However, there is no refrigerator in the room, the vending machines in the hallway have only sodas, and the hotel restaurant closes at 9:00 P.M. After several days alone in the hotel room, Garrett has begun to miss the company of friends and family. He is happy when the week is over.

Many older people who must give up their homes and move into a long-term care facility may feel as if they are living in a hotel room or, even worse, a hospital room, and this experience certainly lasts much longer than a week. In long-term care facilities, the quality and quantity of roles and activities for older people can vary depending on the model of care the facility follows. (See Chapter 1 of this volume for additional information on the different models of care.) For example, a long-term care facility that is based on the hospital model often emphasizes the medical needs of older people without regard to their psychosocial needs. Historically, such long-term care facilities have focused only on simple diversions and leisure activities, including basket weaving or bingo, that are geared primarily toward women. Activities and roles that are related to other areas of older people's lives are not always addressed. With little to do and limited activities, most residents become bored and restless.

Similarly, a long-term care setting that is based on the hospitality model may provide few opportunities for older residents to exercise roles previously held or to participate in activities. Most facilities following this model provide domestic services for residents, such as housekeeping and meals, in much the same way in which a hotel caters to its guests. Recreational activities that people might encounter at a resort or a spa while on vacation are usually stressed, as opposed to leisure activities residents may have participated in before moving into a long-term care facility.

Facilities that have embraced the residential model of care have stressed activities that are meaningful. These facilities have tried to provide more opportunities for residents to be engaged and productive. They have also viewed activities more broadly than simply as recreational diversions. They have included domestic activities, such as folding laundry or setting dining tables, in which many residents would have participated in their own homes before relocation. Other domestic activities that are geared more toward male residents, such as raking leaves, are offered as well. In addition, some facilities have established "work areas" to draw on the roles and activities related to residents' previous work situations. This provides the opportunity to retain these familiar roles if residents so desire.

HOW DEMENTIA AFFECTS ROLES AND ACTIVITIES

Dementia can profoundly affect older people's ability to hold onto roles and to participate in activities. In the early stage, older people may experience some loss of memory, orientation, judgment, and problem-solving skills, and they may have a shorter attention span and a deficit in concentration. They may have trouble remembering the steps that are involved in an activity and the logical sequence of those steps. All of these impairments can prevent older people with dementia from completing complex everyday activities such as balancing a checkbook or following a recipe. Older people with dementia also may fear getting lost, which may discourage them from participating in activities outside their homes. In addition, the inability to control socially inappropriate behaviors, such as vocalizing or disrobing in public, can be a source of embarrassment and can discourage participation in activities involving other people. (Chapter 6 in Volume 3 covers this topic in more detail.)

At first, the inability to participate in activities or to function independently may be interpreted by family members, friends, and co-workers as disinterest, depression, or laziness. Many people with early-stage dementia often retain enough social graces to permit them to hide their impairments and look competent during brief interactions. Family members and even staff may place unrealistic demands on older people with dementia as a result, which can cause them to become angry or to withdraw further (Zgola, 1990). In addition, even when older people with dementia are not entirely aware of their impairments, they sense negativity from their family members and friends. This may cause them to avoid activities and interactions even more. When deficits finally become clear to family members and co-workers, older people with dementia may be forced to give up certain roles such as employee or certain activities such as cooking. This can be extremely upsetting. Imagine how you would feel if you were told that you were making too many mistakes on the job—mistakes of which you were not even aware—and were fired.

As the dementing illness progresses, impaired cognitive skills may prevent older people from performing other tasks that are related to routine self-care, such as dressing, eating, and going to the bathroom. Family members, friends, and caregivers may feel that they must intervene and may restrict all activity for safety reasons or for the person's "own good." Despite the dementia, however, personhood remains. Even in the late stage, older people with dementia retain emotional capacity and attempt to connect with people and objects through touch. They also retain their long-term memory and may be interested in activities, such as baking, that were important to them during their lives. In addition, there is some indication that the need to be productive persists.

Even in the severely demented we continue to see activity—what may appear from the outside to be totally purposeless and repetitive activity: ceaselessly rubbing the chair tray; wringing the hands over and over, hour after hour; perpetually pacing the same route over and over. . . . This speaks to me of the persisting need to do; the desperation to continue activity, even when neurological and physical deficits stand in the way of independent adult activity. (Bowlby, 1993, pp. 84–85)

WHAT STAFF CAN DO

Staff can help in a number of ways to increase opportunities for residents to engage in activities and help residents to retain roles that were previously held before moving into long-term care. Some of these suggestions involve providing appropriate activities for residents related to many areas—domestic, work, and leisure—of their lives. Other recommendations are provided to help direct-care staff or activities programming staff to make activities work. In all cases, administration must fully support staff if these recommendations are to be implemented successfully. In addition, volunteers should be used to the greatest extent possible.

It is also important to note that this volume is not meant to be an activities resource guide. It provides the reader with some ideas to support the roles and activities from older adults' previous home experiences. Several books are available that provide more specific recommendations related to activities programming (Bowlby, 1993; Hellen, 1992; Nissenboim & Vroman, 1997; Zgola, 1987). In addition, "Where to Find Products" includes a list of manufacturers that provide information on or supply activities and activities programming.

Providing Appropriate Activities

Little conclusive research has been done concerning appropriate activities for people with dementia, and it is difficult to make assumptions about what residents like or dislike and whether they are having a good time. To provide appropriate activities for residents, it is necessary first to gather information about each resident's history. Based on this information, activities should be selected that will allow residents to draw on past roles and experiences. It is important to match residents with appropriate activities rather than to fit them into established programs or to rely on stereotypes such as the ubiquitous sing-along (Coons, 1991).

Gathering Information About Each Resident's History

Staff should gather information about each resident's personal history. Although observation of residents certainly can help staff to determine residents' preferences with respect to activities and routines, staff should consider other ways to learn as much as possible about each resident's hobbies and recreational activities; previous occupations; domestic interests; habits; personal accomplishments; religious affiliations and involvement; previous homes and locations; and relationships with parents, children, siblings, and friends. This information is necessary to understand residents as parents, spouses, workers, friends, gardeners, war veterans, artists, and the like. Ideally, staff will gain a greater understanding of who residents were and are as individuals, how they lived in their previous homes, what roles remain important to them, and the activities in which they participated in the past. This information also will help staff to view residents as people in the context of a whole life and will demonstrate that staff care about residents as individuals. More meaningful relationships between staff and residents may result. In addition, staff will be able to involve residents more effectively in appropriate activities that reaffirm the value of their life experiences.

Staff can gather information in a variety of ways. The ideal means of gathering information about individuals who are about to move into a long-term care setting is to have staff visit with potential residents in their current homes and neighborhoods. By observing significant personal possessions in older people's homes and becoming familiar with their patterns of living and places that they have frequented in the community, staff can gain a greater sense of the person as an individual. If this not possible, then ask family members to take pictures or to make a videotape of the person's home before it is disassembled. (Showing these pictures to residents with dementia after they move into the long-term care facility may be therapeutic and may help them to remember their previous homes and experiences. Be aware, however, that some residents may not recognize the places captured in these images, and viewing them may even cause distress for a few. Watch residents carefully to ensure that these images have a positive impact.)

On admission of a new resident, staff should use admission forms that include a sufficient amount of space for documenting personal history and activity interests. Under the Omnibus Budget Reconciliation Act of 1987, nursing facilities certified by Medicare and Medicaid must conduct an assessment of residents' functional abilities, including their activities potential (Perschbacher, 1991, cited in Bowlby, 1993), to ensure quality of life with respect to activities. Questions regarding roles and activities should address multiple areas—domestic, work, and leisure—of each resident's life. Family members may have to provide some assistance with responses to questions. They also may have to help staff determine which interests and roles from which portions of the resident's past are most appropriate. In addition, staff should consider collecting some admission information a second time several weeks after the initial relocation shock. This information likely will be more in depth and will show residents and family members that staff do care about residents as individuals. (Examples of forms for collecting information about residents' histories are included in Appendix A of this volume.)

Staff can gather information about residents who are already living in long-term care settings by meeting with residents and family members and asking about each resident's history. In the process, the importance of providing activities that relate to the resident's previous interests and roles can be emphasized. To document the information gathered from these sessions, family members can be encouraged to write a one-page description of the resident's history. Research has shown that staff who read a one-page personal history in residents' medical charts learned more about the residents and viewed them more positively than did staff who were not provided with residents' personal histories in medical charts (Petrukowicz & Johnson, 1991, cited in Bowlby, 1993). Thus, personal histories are important, and staff should be provided with the necessary time to review these documents. They also should be encouraged to share this information with one another. In addition, activities staff should consider keeping this information in a portable binder for easy reference. This information should remain confidential, to be used by staff only in a discrete manner.

Often, this type of information can be useful in dealing with residents who exhibit challenging behaviors. Most people do what they do for a reason. For residents with dementia, however, caregivers may have a difficult time determining what that reason is and developing a strategy to manage the behavior. For example, a resident may be combative during a domestic activity such as folding laundry. If it is not clear why a resident is combative, then it may be helpful to use a behavior tracking process during which staff can record some basic information each time the behavior occurs to understand the behavior. Staff should record the 5 Ws—who, what (e.g., what behavior), where, when, and why. The 5 Ws are

- Who—the name of the resident
- What—what is the resident doing and what is happening on the unit
- Where—where did the behavior occur
- When—what time it is
- Why—why you think the resident behaved this way

Although a number of factors may be causing the combative behavior, staff may discover that it is because the resident with dementia was used to having a housekeeper and never enjoyed domestic activities. (Volume 3, Chapter 1 covers behavior tracking in more detail. A behavior tracking form that can be used for the tracking process is provided in Appendix A in that volume.)

Identifying Activities from Three Areas of Life

Once the resident's history has been documented, staff should identify activities that permit the continuation of lifelong roles and interests. Emphasis should be placed on familiar activities from the three areas of residents' lives—domestic, work, and leisure—that are embedded in long-term memory. A balance of all three areas is essential to well-being. These activities also should be authentic to the greatest extent possible. Residents in the early and middle stages of dementia, for instance, may be able to clip coupons from daily newspapers. Rather than being thrown away, these coupons can be used by staff or visiting family members. Residents also can participate in volunteer activities. If the facility has mailings to prepare, then residents can help fold brochures and stuff and stamp envelopes. Such activities become meaningful instead of merely being diversions that are used to fill up a day and keep residents "out of their hair."

The facility should offer familiar domestic activities such as food preparation, table setting, and cleanup because many older women currently living in long-term care facilities were homemakers. This is easier to do when residents have access to a small kitchen (discussed further in "What the Environment Can Do"). If small therapeutic kitchens do not exist in the facility, then residents can still help by setting tables in the dining room at mealtimes or by participating in other domestic activities such as folding laundry or dusting furniture. Staff can provide supervision or some guidance if necessary. Whether these activities are done correctly is not important; it is only important that residents remain involved. What residents think and feel is useful and productive is more important than what staff view as productive.

> Millie followed a nursing assistant around the dementia-specific care unit, entering bedrooms and unmaking beds as soon as the aide left the bedrooms after making the beds. When the nursing assistant discovered this, she was ready to scream. After watching and tracking the behavior for a while, staff noticed how content Millie was while unmaking beds. She thought she was being helpful and was very proud of her work. Staff realized that this reflected Millie's need to be productive and to contribute to the upkeep of her living environment. Instead of trying to prevent her from engaging in the behavior, the nursing assistant invited Millie to help her as she made the beds. It took longer, but not as long as it took to go back and remake all of the beds. With a little direction, Millie was able to start making the beds on her own while the nursing assistant straightened other parts of the room.

Staff also should recognize that domestic activities are not appropriate for everyone. Although most of the women in this cohort were probably homemakers, some may not have enjoyed this role or the activities that are associated with taking care of a home. Others may have had maids and were not accustomed to engaging in these types of activities. In other words, it is important to realize that one solution is not appropriate for everyone; it is necessary to consider the various life experiences of different social classes of the older adult population in relation to domestic activities (Marsden, 1993).

Domestic activities take place outside the home as well. For example, the facility can incorporate gardening in an activity program. (This topic is discussed in greater detail in "What the Environment Can Do.") Flowers that result from gardening activities can be used for flower arranging, with residents making small centerpieces for dining room tables. Other outdoor domestic activities that involve physical work, such as raking leaves or sweeping patios, may appeal to some of the men in the facility. Men in this cohort were often responsible for taking care of the outsides of their homes, yet indoor activities that are geared primarily toward women are usually all that are provided in long-term care facilities. Staff may find that some "typically male" activities may be preferred by some of the women in the facility as well.

The facility should provide work-oriented activities in addition to domestic activities. Most of the men and some of the women living in long-term care settings were part of the workforce at one time. Work may have been a significant part of their lives and a source from which they could derive a sense of productivity and usefulness. This part of the past lives of residents with dementia may be more salient than their current situation. Thus, it is important to draw on past work experiences. Reminiscing about work individually with a caregiver or as part of a group discussion is one way to tap into this part of residents' lives. Another way is to set up a work area, such as a desk with a typewriter. Residents can fold facility brochures or file papers at this desk. If a resident was a carpenter, then a safe woodworking area can be established where the resident can sand and varnish a piece of furniture or a small wooden toy for children (see "What the Environment Can Do" later in this chapter).

Leisure and recreational activities typically have been the focus of most activity programs in long-term care settings. To appeal to the wide variety of interests and life experiences of the residents, staff should offer many different kinds of leisure activities. These can include passive activities such as watching movies or travelogues; more active activities such as flower arranging, dancing, or playing boccie; structured activities such as bingo; and unstructured activities such as visiting with a pet. Outings are important as well.

At one facility, a "lunch bunch" was formed for residents who were interested in going out to lunch. With a staff member's help, residents in this group identify different restaurants in the community through advertisements in newspapers and magazines. Residents talk about their food preferences and select three different restaurants for a particular day. Some residents like to go to the food court at the mall or a cafe in the middle of town, while others prefer certain chain restaurants in which they used to eat before moving into the long-term care facility. The facility provides transportation, and four to six residents go to each of the three restaurants. Depending on the selection of restaurants, various people join the lunch bunch on different days. On the way back to the facility, residents often talk about their meals as well as other restaurants they would like to go to in the future. Residents look forward to these lunch outings so much that the lunch bunch, with the facility's help, ventures out about three times per week.

Trips into the community, such as shopping at the mall, visiting a park, or attending a concert, provide a sense of normality for residents. In all cases, leisure activities should have a purpose, whether it is relaxation, entertainment, or exercise. For example, walking in a mall from store to store to buy a birthday gift for a grandchild is much more meaningful than walking around a circular pathway over and over again to satisfy physical therapy requirements.

Making the Activities Work

Once staff have gathered sufficient background information about residents and have used this information to identify appropriate activities, several strategies can be used to make these activities work. These strategies include providing activities at which residents can succeed, using techniques to sustain participation, providing reality validation, encouraging participation rather than enforcing it, and providing adult activities.

Providing Activities at Which Residents Can Succeed

To provide activities at which residents can succeed, staff should consider activities that draw on the strengths and remaining abilities of residents. Thus, it is important for staff to know who the residents are as individuals. Providing one resident with a crossword puzzle may be frustrating if he or she is somewhat of a perfectionist and can no longer do this activity. In contrast, another resident may be content to carry around the puzzle, asking others to help out as needed.

Drawing on overlearned, familiar skills is another way in which residents can succeed while participating in activities (Zgola, 1990). For instance, a resident who spent most of his working life as a gardener could be asked to take care of two or three plants in the facility. With guidance and reminders from staff, he could be responsible for pruning and watering the plants. Similarly, asking a resident to serve tea and cookies can draw on familiar social skills that remind her of her role as a charming hostess.

Success also can result when residents participate in activities that are virtually failure free (Bowlby, 1993). Asking a resident to do something as simple as folding laundry, in which there really is not a correct procedure or outcome, can provide residents with a sense of accomplishment. Some residents may be content to fold the same towels repeatedly. Others may not and will need other things to fold as well, such as napkins for meals. Providing music is another possibility. Residents with dementia can appreciate and respond to music; the parts of the brain that are involved in this activity usually are not damaged by dementia. Some residents simply may tap their feet to the music, while others may want to dance or play musical instruments. Music provides opportunities for a range of responses.

In addition, activities and roles that involve past positive experiences may result in success (Zgola, 1990). Reminiscing about a resident's positive experiences fixing cars, for example, may sustain his attention because the reminiscence reminds him of something he was able to do well. When such activities provide immediate feedback, there is a greater chance for success (Zgola, 1990). Low-functioning residents will have a harder time trying to express desired activities and roles. In such cases, staff should draw on roles that are enduring regardless of the stage of dementia. For example, being a friend, telling residents that they are good friends, and treating them like friends can be beneficial.

Using Techniques to Sustain Participation

Several techniques can be used to sustain participation in activities. First, staff should keep activities simple. As few verbal instructions as possible should be required, and decisions that must be made by residents should be within their skill levels. Activities that involve the same step over and over again, such as dusting furniture, are ideal. Otherwise, staff may have to provide step-by-step guidance. If multiple steps are involved, then staff should make sure that the first step of the activity will lead to success. Activities that do not demand long attention spans or good coordination are also beneficial (Gwyther, 1985). Second, staff should not use activities that require new skills or learning. This can be disheartening and discouraging for residents. Activities should draw on overlearned skills and patterns of behavior embedded in long-term memory. For example, a resident who played piano for many years before moving into a long-term care facility may be able to sit down and play a favorite song from memory if she sees a piano in an activity room. However, the same resident may not be able to learn from sheet music a new song that someone else might want to hear. Third, structured activities involving small groups or one-to-one interaction tend to work better with residents with cognitive impairment than do unstructured activities such as painting (Zgola, 1990). Fourth, staff should avoid activities that involve asking questions. Questions that require precise answers or open-ended questions will only expose impairments (Zgola, 1990) and remind residents that they cannot remember things or take care of themselves. One way to avoid this is to provide activities that emphasize nonverbal skills, such as petting a dog. Fifth, staff should consider including one or two high-functioning residents in group activities. These residents can serve as models and as stimuli for other residents (Bowlby, 1993).

Providing Reality Orientation

A number of long-term care facilities use activities that involve orienting residents to time, date, and place, or reality orientation. Reality orientation has been used to orient residents with dementia. This involves providing correct information to residents who are confused about their current situation. Telling a resident that her husband is deceased when she talks about him coming for a visit is one example. The advisability of orienting residents to the present is a debatable topic. In general, staff should proceed with caution when using traditional reality orientation with residents with dementia.

Some residents with mild to moderate cognitive impairments may ask staff for orientation cues, and should be provided with accurate information. However, it is probably not effective to train these residents to remember facts such as dates and times. As the cognitive impairment that is associated with dementia increases, reality orientation sometimes can do more damage than good. Telling residents with more severe impairment 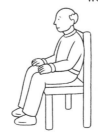 something other than what they believe to be true may only frighten or upset them. For instance, telling a woman with dementia that her husband is dead may cause her to relive the whole grieving process, resulting in a lot of unnecessary pain. (Volume 2, Chapter 2 covers reality orientation in more detail.)

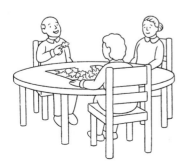

Do Not Force Participation

Staff should realize that many residents may not wish to participate in activities. Some residents may have been loners or may have high privacy needs (see Chapter 4 of this volume for additional information). In these instances, residents should not be forced to participate in activities; participation always should be voluntary. Sometimes, however, residents may need gentle persuasion. It is not uncommon, for instance, for residents with dementia to turn down invitations to participate in activities because they fear embarrassment or exposure of their impairments. Staff should suggest to these residents that they can watch the activity in progress first and then ease into the activity as they feel more comfortable (Zgola, 1990). In addition, residents can be paired up with a "friend" so that they do not have to attend the activity alone. As is true of most social situations, it is easier to participate if you know someone else who is going to be at the activity.

Providing Adult Activities

If activities are childlike or are perceived that way by residents, then the long-term care setting can present an image to staff and family members that residents are indeed like children. This can result in care that reinforces dependency. Providing residents with coloring books and large-piece children's puzzles or asking them to make holiday decorations out of construction paper are examples of childlike activities. There are times, however, when activities that may be perceived as childlike by others are actually therapeutic. For instance, a resident may have collected teddy bears as an adult. Taking care of these teddy bears and carrying them around the facility may help to comfort him or her. In this case, it is important to understand the previous interests of the resident as an adult and to encourage those interests. In contrast, providing residents with teddy bears to cuddle when they did not engage in such behavior before moving into the facility does not reflect their adult status. Because there may be some residents who do enjoy some of these more child-oriented activities, these types of activities should, whenever possible, involve interactions with children from the community. In other words, it is appropriate for residents to use crayons or to cut out construction paper in a joint activity with children.

WHAT THE ENVIRONMENT CAN DO

This section offers ideas for creating or modifying spaces that support roles and activities from various areas of residents' lives. These ideas include suggestions for indoor spaces, such as therapeutic kitchens, and outdoor spaces, such as courtyards and garden areas, that can support domestic activities. Ideas also are provided that address work stations to support work-related activities as well as indoor and outdoor spaces for leisure activities.

Domestic Activities

Taking care of a home, both inside and outside, is something that most of us do throughout our lifetimes. For many older adults living in long-term care settings, especially women, the ability to continue participating in domestic activities helps to reinforce their previous roles. A therapeutic kitchen in a long-term care setting can serve as the site for such activity. At the same time, outdoor spaces that support domestic activities traditionally geared more toward men are also important.

Therapeutic Kitchens

The kitchen is often the center of a home. For many older women, the kitchen is a familiar and comfortable environment. Providing a small therapeutic kitchen for residents to use may help them draw on familiar routines, roles, and patterns of behavior. Washing dishes, setting tables, sweeping floors, folding laundry, cleaning vegetables, and decorating cookies are a few of the activities that can take place in a therapeutic kitchen. At the same time, a therapeutic kitchen can be the site of informal gatherings and socialization. While people are working together, the domestic activities can provide a common topic for conversation that promotes socialization (Figure 3.1).

Creating a therapeutic kitchen can be accomplished even if the facility does not have a place for cabinets, a counter, a sink, a stove, or a refrigerator. If the facility is in a rural area or many of the residents were farmers or grew up on farms, then consider adding a large farmhouse-type table for casual gatherings of six to eight people in a kitchen area. If residents have a more urban or suburban background, the facility should consider a different type of kitchen table. In general, a table can provide a focus for and enhance socialization. Smaller worktables with seating, a baker's rack, and an old cupboard are a few of the items you can add to a kitchen area. The kitchen can be accessorized with a canister set, potholders, a bread box, or other familiar, noninstitutional items that residents would normally find in their homes. These items provide cues for the types of activities that can take place in the space. In addition, a storage space for brooms and dust rags would be necessary, and a sink would be beneficial.

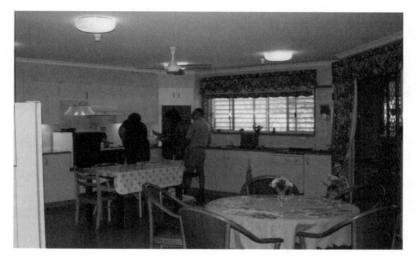

Figure 3.1. A therapeutic kitchen can provide opportunities for socialization while giving residents a place to participate in domestic activities.

Where space permits, the facility can consider adding other appliances in the kitchen area. Refrigerators can be used for storing snacks. Stoves can provide many wonderful aromas but also raise safety concerns. Should a stove be added, it should have a hidden power switch that automatically turns the appliance off after a certain amount of time. You should check with the local fire marshal about restrictions before incorporating a stove within a kitchen area. If a stove cannot be added, then cookie jars, popcorn popping, or coffee brewing can provide aroma cues. A washer and dryer can be added as well. The washer and dryer should be grouped together in an area that is located away from the kitchen appliances to minimize confusion.

Outdoor Spaces

In their lives before the nursing facility, many older men were responsible for taking care of the outsides of their homes and may wish to continue these patterns of behavior. The facility should provide outdoor spaces that support domestic activities such as raking leaves, sweeping pathways, weeding, and planting vegetables. If there is enough space, then secure front and backyards surrounded by a fence and accessible from the building can be provided. Taking care of a lawn or maintaining foundation shrubs may be appropriate activities for a front yard, whereas planting vegetables may be something residents can do in a backyard. In all cases, gardening areas should be raised or tall flowers should be planted so that residents do not have to stoop or bend over too often. (See "Where to Find Products" for a source of raised garden beds. Appendix C of this volume presents a list of toxic plants to avoid.) The facility should provide seating throughout the garden in case residents need to rest periodically, places for shade, and a lockable storage shed for work supplies.

Outdoor spaces that support activities that are geared toward female residents are important as well. The facility can provide gardening areas and an old-fashioned clothesline near the building for hanging laundry. A patio space that is large enough can support a tea party or an ice cream social. Tables and chairs and a serving table would be necessary (see "Where to Find Products"). Residents can help serve the tea or ice cream. In addition, the facility should consider adding play areas for children. Swings, slides, and a sandbox can be used by visiting grandchildren or by children in the community if they are brought for a visit.

Work Activities

For most of the men and some of the women living in long-term care settings, paid work was a source of productivity, usefulness, and meaning. Setting up work areas and workshops in the facility is beneficial to support these kinds of activities for high-functioning residents. Creating places to rummage may also help low-functioning residents to feel productive.

Work Areas

A work area can provide residents with a place to go to work. Desks and office chairs may be appropriate props and cues for residents who previously worked in office environments. The facility can add accessories such as typewriters, reading lamps, writing pads, pens, and file folders. Typewriters that would have been used when residents actually were employed might be more beneficial for residents with memory impairment than modern typewriters or computers. Similarly, the facility can create a grandmother's corner for residents who took care of their families in the home. This area can be as simple as a rocking chair and a small set of shelves with children's books and soft toys. Families might feel more comfortable about bringing children to long-term care settings if they know that the children will have things to play with while on the unit. The facility can establish these productive work areas within a portion of a resident's bedroom, in an activity room, or near a staff station because residents often like to be where the action is.

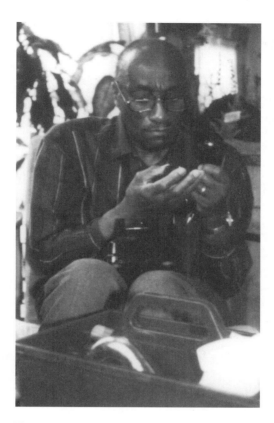

Figure 3.2. A table and chair, tools, and some small parts will allow a resident who was a telephone repairman to assemble and disassemble equipment.

Workshops

Work areas can be set aside for residents who were involved in occupations such as carpentry or plumbing. These areas can be temporary, inside or outside the building. A small table and a chair may be all that is needed. For example, a resident who previously worked as a carpenter could work at an outdoor table on a patio. The table can be protected with newspaper from sawdust, paint, and varnish. A resident who worked as a telephone repairman could be provided with tools and small parts that can be put together and then taken apart while the resident is seated at a table (Figure 3.2). Similarly, someone who worked in a floral shop may only need a table, access to water, dried or fresh flowers, and a couple of vases to work happily on flower arrangements for hours.

Places to Rummage

Residents who engage in rummaging may be looking for things to do or may be seeking tactile stimulation. To satisfy these needs, staff should consider providing appropriate places to rummage in various parts of the facility. Some residents may prefer to be closer to staff and to feel a part of the productive life of the unit. This suggests a location close to the nurses' station or other activity center. Others may prefer to be more secretive about their rummaging and stay in their rooms (or wander into others' rooms). In such cases, rummaging areas can be provided in more remote corners of the unit. Places to rummage can include chests of drawers (Figure 3.3) or boxes filled with a variety of objects with different tactile qualities placed in lounges or activity rooms. (See "Where to Find Products" for sources of supplies for creating rummaging areas.) Eventually, residents realize that there are places where they can always find something interesting to touch, look at, or do. Other places to rummage can include bookshelves in a lounge or living room that contain books and knickknacks that can be straightened and organized over and over again. (Volume 3, Chapter 4 covers rummaging and hoarding in more detail.)

Leisure Activities

Spaces also can be modified in various ways to support leisure activities. Furniture arrangements, opportunities for personalization, and the division of large spaces into smaller, less overwhelming ones can help. Many of these principles are appropriate for both the inside and outside of a facility. Spaces can be created for specific activities as well.

Furniture Arrangements

When conducting small group activities, a table can serve as a focus for socialization. The table should be accessible to everyone, including those using wheelchairs or geri-chairs. Residents who are compatible should be placed beside each other, while those who are most disruptive should be placed at the ends of the table (Bowlby, 1993). In addition, a table can serve as a place for props and supplies. Staff should have these items readily available before beginning the activity.

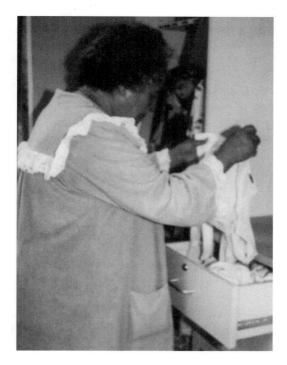

Figure 3.3. Special drawers can be constructed to provide residents with opportunities for rummaging and sorting.

For smaller group activities that do not require a table, seating should be arranged at right angles to facilitate communication between residents and staff. Chairs arranged around the perimeter of a room are not particularly welcoming. For those residents who are hesitant about participating in activities and would like to watch first, a few single chairs along the perimeter of the space can be provided.

Opportunities for Personalization

Personalization is important in all parts of the facility, from private bedrooms to shared spaces such as living rooms (see Chapter 2 in this volume). Familiar items such as knickknacks, furniture from previous homes, and pictures can be added to spaces in the facility and used for reminiscing or for actual activities. For example, a quilt that a resident with dementia made for one of her daughters can remind her of her relationship with her child and can encourage her to crochet other items (in the early stage of dementia) or simply to touch balls of yarn (in the late stage).

If residents or family members do not wish to place personal belongings in shared spaces, then residential-looking vintage items that might spark past memories can be used instead. An old radio, for instance, may remind residents of times when they sat with their families to listen to the news. A trunk filled with old hats and clothes may encourage some residents to try on different outfits. Similarly, seasonal decorations that typically would be encountered in residents' previous homes are important for orienting residents and encouraging participation in holiday activities. For example, residents can help decorate a Christmas tree in the living room of the facility.

Division of Space

Certain group activities are more successful when there are fewer distractions. One way to make interior spaces more manageable is to divide large spaces into smaller, less overwhelming ones. The facility can accomplish this with furniture and folding partition walls (refer to "Where to Find Products" for sources). These allow flexibility because spaces can be divided and opened up depending on the activity that is taking place. A more permanent solution is to build half-walls, possibly with glass above them, to differentiate space and allow some visibility between areas. This is desirable for residents who wish to watch activities before making a commitment to participate. Outdoor spaces can be divided into smaller areas with outdoor furniture, including tables and chairs and porch swings, garden planters, retaining walls, and landscaping.

Creation of Spaces with Themes

In addition to leisure activities that take place within individual homes, people often pursue activities within the community. Spaces can be created within a facility that replicates places residents may have frequented before relocating. For example, a room on a hallway can be turned into a soda shop by opening up the wall that faces the hallway, using the name and decor of a well-known shop in the community, placing a couple of small tables with chairs in the space, and serving soda and ice cream. (Check state codes to determine whether you can open up the wall facing the hallway.) These types of spots often serve as gathering places when families come to visit. Some facilities have small nooks or recessed areas of hallways that can be creatively used instead. One facility created a barber shop by building a half-wall with red-and-white striped barber poles (Figure 3.4). Residents immediately were able to

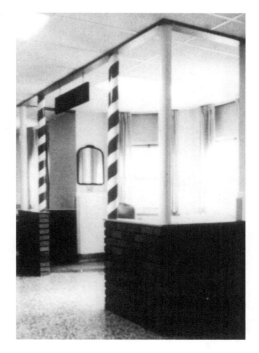

Figure 3.4.   The construction of a half-wall with striped poles provided residents with a "barber shop" where they could sit and converse.

identify it as the place where they went to get a shave. A few chairs within were all that was needed for residents to stop and chat as they did in their own community barber shop. These types of changes may trigger memories of past places and encourage socialization.

WHERE TO FIND PRODUCTS

Activities and Activity Programming

AARP Sources
601 E Street NW
Washington, DC 20049
(800) 424-3410

American Historic Society
Accessible through *www.SkyMall.com*
A variety of old-time products, including bulk packages of unopened baseball cards

Briggs Corporation
7300 Westown Parkway
West Des Moines, IA 50266
(800) 247-2343
www.briggscorp.com
A variety of activity products, including a bowling alley carpet and pins

Eymann Publications, Inc.
Post Office Box 3577
Reno, NV 89505
(800) 354-3371
www.care4elders.com
Publisher of the newsletter *Activity Director's Guide*

Geriatric Resources, Inc.
11636 North Dona Ana Road
Las Cruces, NM 88005
(800) 359-0390
www.geriatric-resources.com
Publishes a catalog of activity-related products and games

The Haworth Press
10 Alice Street
Binghamton, NY 13904-1580
(800) 342-9678
www.haworthpressinc.com
Publishes *Activities, Adaptation and Aging,* a quarterly journal that provides practical research on activity programming

Innovative Caregiving Resources
Post Office Box 17809
Salt Lake City, UT 84117-0809
(800) 249-5600
www.videorespite.com
Activity programs using videotapes

Leisure and Aging Publications
2775 South Quincy Street, Suite 300
Arlington, VA 22206-2204
A catalog of activity-related publications

NASCO
901 Janesville Avenue
Post Office Box 901
Fort Atkinson, WI 53538-0901
(800) 558-9595
www.enasco.com
Publishes a catalog of activity programming products

Potentials
40 Hazelwood Drive, Suite 101
Amherst, NY 14228
(800) 691-6602
A catalog of activity programming targeted to activity directors

United Seniors Health Cooperative
409 Third Street SW, Suite 200
Washington, DC 20024
(202) 479-6973
www.unitedseniorshealth.org
Eldergames trivia books and picture card sets

Companion Radio
1 Fisher Road
Pittsford, NY 14534
(800) 499-4040
A satellite radio program featuring age-appropriate programming

Sound Choice
14100 South Lakes Drive
Charlotte, NC 28273
(888) 465-4400
www.soundchoice.com
Reminiscing series—karaoke featuring music from 1900 to the 1940s

Gardening

StandUp Gardens, Ltd.
34 Patterson Lane
Portsmouth, NH 03801
(800) TO-STAND
www.standupgardens.com
A portable gardening area that can be used indoors or out, does not require residents to stoop, and provides a gardening experience for residents with various capabilities.

Outdoor Furniture

Fincastle County Chairworks
2821 South English Station Road
Louisville, KY 40299
(502) 267-1888
Resin furniture that looks like wood but will not deteriorate

Leisure Woods
Post Office Box 177
Genoa, IL 60135
(800) 422-9326

Marin Deck Chair
230 Arroyo Road
Lagunitas, CA 94938-0294
(415) 488-4477
www.sunorshade.com
Chaise de Soleil outdoor glider

WhisperGLIDE
10051 Kerry Court
Hugo, MN 55038
(800) 944-7737
www.whisperglide.com
WhisperGLIDE outdoor glider swing

Creating Rummaging Areas

Exposures, Inc.
Post Office Box 3615
Oshkosh, WI 54903-3615
(800) 222-4947
www.exposuresonline.com
A catalog of items for the storage and display of photographs and mementos

Hold Everything
Post Office Box 7807
San Francisco, CA 94120-7807
(800) 421-2264
www.holdeverything.com
A catalog featuring storage items

JC Penney
(800) 222-6161
Offers a variety of unfinished, easy-to-assemble furniture that can become activity projects for residents

Cabinets for Dividing Dining Rooms

Adden Furniture, Inc.
26 Jackson Street
Lowell, MA 01852
(508) 457-7848

Allsteel, Inc.
Allsteel Drive
Aurora, IL 60507
(800) 764-2535
www.allsteeloffice.com
Their InterChange System panel system consists of dividers with
acoustical inserts on both sides. The company also offers a variety of
wheeled cabinets for storage.

◆◆◆

A summary sheet follows, which condenses the chapter text into a
quick overview. The authors have also provided an area for you to make your
own notes about your own staff and facility. Managerial staff may wish to use
the summary sheets as handouts to accompany direct care staff training, or to
post them by the time clock or nurses' station or include them in staff's pay
envelopes.

ROLES AND ACTIVITIES SUMMARY SHEET

1. People are often defined by their roles (e.g., grandmother, husband, librarian, waitress, construction worker).

2. Our roles affect what we do (our activities) and who we interact with.

3. Roles affect feelings of self-worth. (Think of how people who are out of work feel, or the slogan "Proud to be a Marine.")

4. People lose many of these roles when they relocate into a long-term care setting. Many try to recreate these roles (e.g., the resident who finds a "new" wife) because they lose connection with their old roles and relationships.

What Staff Can Do

1. Determine what roles and relationships were important to each resident. This includes, work, domestic, and leisure roles.

2. Find activities to support these roles in residents' new residence and lifestyle. Examples include daily housekeeping or household chores, regular opportunities for familiar hobbies (e.g., going out to lunch, bowling weekly), and opportunities to contribute productively (e.g., fold and stuff envelopes, work on a small engine or telephone).

3. Structure activities for residents so that they are failure-free.

4. Be a friend to each resident.

5. Create individual work baskets or boxes for each resident based on their previous interests.

What the Environment Can Do

1. Provide places (e.g., kitchen, shop, office) for different kinds of familiar activities.

YOUR NOTES

4
Privacy

Privacy can mean many things to different people. For some, it means being alone. For others, it means maintaining a certain physical distance while talking. It also can mean not being seen in your bathrobe, not being overheard, or not being the subject of neighborhood gossip. In all cases, privacy is the ability to regulate what you reveal about yourself, through sight, sound, touch, and access to thoughts, as well as what information you receive from others. Privacy also involves the ability to control social contact. In other words, there are instances in which people do not want to interact with others and there are times when interaction is welcomed. Privacy is important for many reasons. In private, you can let your hair down, take a step back and reflect on what is happening in your life, and control what you reveal about yourself to others. The ability to protect information about yourself and your life is important as well.

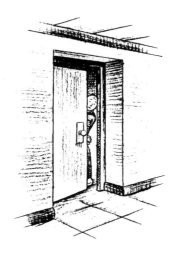

LETTING YOUR HAIR DOWN

How many times have you felt so excited about something that you wished you could have yelled out loud in a shopping mall or in the middle of a street? Suppose you just received news while you are at work that your sister is pregnant. You might have wanted to jump up and down but felt that would be inappropriate in the office. Or you may have just seen a very sad and moving film that touched you. You may have prevented yourself from crying in the theater, especially if you are a man, largely because society discourages public emotional displays. This behavior is permitted only under certain circumstances, such as at funerals. After leaving the theater, you may have experienced additional embarrassment if you walked into a diner for something to eat and found yourself among people who would consider you odd for carrying on in public because they did not see the same sad movie. In other words, there are times when people need privacy to display their true emotions and to relieve themselves of the various roles they feel that they must assume in public.

People often are like actors on a dramatic stage (Goffman, 1956). As actors, however, we can role-play only for certain periods of time before demanding relief. Relief is usually sought "offstage," out of the public eye, where people can remove their masks, let their hair down, and truly be themselves without having to meet expected behaviors and norms.

> *Jim is sitting at his desk reading the morning newspaper when he notices his boss approaching his cubicle with someone he does not recognize. Jim quickly hides his newspaper and tries to look like he is engrossed in his work. When his boss reaches the cubicle, she explains that she is giving a tour to a prospective employee. She introduces Jim and asks him how he likes working for the company. Jim forces a smile and replies that he feels lucky to be working for such a good organization. As soon as his boss leaves, Jim peers over his cubicle to talk to Erin, who sits next to him. "I would have really liked to tell the new hire that our boss is very controlling and that this company expects us to work too much overtime," says Jim. Bill, who sits across from Jim, joins in before Erin can respond. "I hear you. My wife wants to know when I'm going to start helping out around the house more with the laundry and the kids. I keep telling her that all this overtime is killing me." When Jim gets home that evening, he tells his wife about his boss and how the company is not supportive. He also tells her about how Bill uses work as an excuse so that he does not have to spend as much time with his kids.*

In this example, Jim assumed the role of a diligent, content employee when his boss passed by his cubicle, even though he is unhappy with his work environment. He was able to let his hair down a little bit around Erin and Bill, his co-workers. In the privacy of his own home, out of the public eye and offstage, Jim was able to talk freely with his wife about his boss, the company, and his co-workers.

Many people have a particular offstage place to which they retreat for privacy. For example, one individual may locks him- or herself in a bathroom for peace and quiet. Alternatively, other people feel a sense of privacy when they are lost in the crowd of a large city or a busy shopping mall.

SELF-REFLECTION

While relaxing in private offstage, we have the chance to review and make sense of all of the things that have happened to us that day or during the week. This is rather difficult to do while onstage, where we are constantly bombarded with information. For example, have you ever found yourself so busy with your children—getting them ready for school, checking their homework, chauffeuring them to soccer practice or to a friend's house, and cooking them dinner—that you have not had a chance to take a step back and evaluate how you are changing as a result of your relationship with your children? Many of us put so much energy into our children that we simply do not have time for self-reflection. Or you may have been so caught up in a new love relationship that you spent most of your free time with your partner. You may have felt that you were losing part of your self in the process. You may have then found it necessary to reflect on your relationship, to determine whether it was affecting you as you would like, and to plan how you should proceed.

In this sense, privacy is an important part of our sense of self. It "allows us the time and space to reflect on the meaning of events, to fit them into our understanding of the world, and to formulate a response to them that is consistent with our self-image" (Gifford, 1997, p. 182). In other words, people need to process information and then plan for the future, and this can be accomplished most effectively in private.

CONTROL

Privacy can also facilitate our sense of control. The ability to choose what we do or do not reveal about ourselves and with whom we interact is linked to control and can vary for different people in various situations. For instance, a Hollywood movie star may not have much control over what personal information is revealed in the tabloids or over fans who may overwhelm him or her in public. However, a wealthy movie star may be able to control, to a degree, other people's access to him or her by being chauffeured in a car with dark, tinted windows so that people cannot see in, by going to exclusive restaurants, and by living in a house in a secluded area with a tall security fence around the property. For most people, privacy is established on a much smaller scale.

> *Lisa and a close friend had been planning to see a movie that had just opened at the theater in their neighborhood. At the last minute, her friend called to say that she would not be able to make it. Lisa was dying to see the movie and decided to go on her own. When Lisa walked inside the theater, she looked around for a seat that had an empty seat on both sides. She had never been to a movie on her own and did not really want to sit next to someone she did not know. She placed her jacket on the seat to her right. A few minutes later, a man sat in the seat to her left. Lisa was surprised because there were other seats available that were farther away. She wished that she had something to put on that seat. She felt uncomfortable and folded her arms. The man then asked her what time it was, and Lisa replied in a cold tone without looking at him. When he asked another question, Lisa grabbed her jacket and moved to another part of the theater. Fortunately, Lisa had some control and was able take action when she felt her personal space was invaded.*

In work situations, people may chat or have lunch with co-workers in a staff break room away from management. Some people may try to find a quiet place somewhere else to sit and have lunch alone. Others may leave the office and go to a deli. While outside, they may make private calls from a pay phone so that they do not have worry about being overheard by co-workers. These are instances in which people control the amount of privacy—information revealed as well as social contact—that they desire at work (see Chapter 5 of this volume for additional information).

PROTECTING INFORMATION ABOUT THE SELF

There are times when people may wish to reveal personal or intimate details about themselves. For example, you may want to discuss a problem you are having in your marriage with a sibling or a close friend you trust. You might hold back some of the details because you consider them too personal or embarrassing, but, in general, you do not mind sharing most of this information.

If you need some comfort, then you probably would not mind if your sibling or friend gave you a hug. In other situations, however, people might not want to reveal such information about themselves. For instance, you probably would not want to discuss your marital troubles with your mother-in-law or your boss. You probably would not feel comfortable hugging the president of the company that employs you or sharing a hotel room with co-workers who usually do not see you in your nightclothes or without your makeup.

The amount of information that people wish to protect can vary depending on their backgrounds. For instance, a person who was raised in a large family may have different privacy needs than someone who grew up in a small family. People from larger families may be used to more intrusions, less space, and the need to share bedrooms and bathrooms. Those who immigrated to the United States from other countries also may have different privacy needs. Survivors of the Holocaust, for example, often experienced conditions in concentration camps in which privacy did not exist. They may have been forced to adapt and now value their privacy even more. In contrast, some cultures do not value privacy; people prefer to be surrounded by family members and find it frightening to be alone.

People can protect information about themselves in several ways. For example, people protect privacy through body gestures. If you ran into someone with whom you did not particularly want to talk, then you might turn your back to the person or use certain facial expressions, such as a scowl, to discourage any sort of interaction. If someone were to ask you inappropriate personal questions you did not want to answer, then you might protect your privacy by changing the tone of your voice, changing the topic of conversation, or exchanging private jokes with someone else present to exclude the person asking the personal questions.

People also protect information about themselves with personal space or what has been referred to as the *invisible bubble* immediately surrounding the self (Sommer, 1966). This personal space stretches and shrinks depending on who is involved in the social interaction; the distance between you and the other person; whether the other person is in front of, behind, or beside you; and the situation or context. Feelings about personal space are often established by society, and people are expected to follow these unwritten rules. For example, according to anthropologist Edward T. Hall, a distance of less than 18 inches is considered an intimate range for interacting with others in North America (cited in Deasy & Lasswell, 1990). People rarely sit next to someone they do not know at a bus stop or in an airport if they have a choice; they like to keep an empty seat between them. Also, people usually consider a hug from a stranger to be a rude invasion of personal space. Nevertheless, there are some instances in which people are willing to allow others to penetrate their personal space, such as when they are in an airplane or an elevator.

In addition, people can protect information about themselves by marking a territory as their own. With respect to their homes, people may try to protect their privacy by marking the property with a fence, installing a dead bolt on the front door, or installing blinds in a picture window overlooking the street. People use all of these methods to help keep unwanted strangers away and to protect themselves from visual observation by nearby neighbors and those passing on the street.

HOW PRIVACY NEEDS CHANGE WITH AGE AND RELOCATION

Throughout life, the need for privacy remains constant. Even as people age, they still need privacy to let their hair down, for self-reflection, to protect information about themselves, and for the opportunity to control social interaction and the amount of information they choose to reveal to others. In the later stages of life, however, older adults may experience too much privacy if their social support network diminishes. They also may desire more privacy when they experience health-related problems or must move into a long-term care facility occupied by people they do not know.

Decreased Social Support

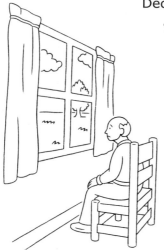

The number of people present in the lives of older adults decreases as they age. All of these losses can result in less social contact and fewer life roles to play (see Chapter 3 of this volume for additional information on this topic). Because these losses usually are not initiated by them and are imposed by uncontrollable circumstances, older adults often find themselves experiencing much more privacy than they would like. This can lead to social and emotional loneliness, which is particularly evident with certain losses, such as the death of a spouse. Not only does the older adult lose the companionship and intimacy of the person to whom he or she was most important but he or she also may have difficulty fitting in with friends who are still part of a couple. Opportunities for interaction with others can be even more difficult in suburban neighborhoods, where older adults are dependent on a car to meet others or to participate in community activities. In addition, some older adults may not see any point in initiating new friendships because they fear additional social losses. Yet research indicates that social support is an important determinant of well-being for older people (Kimmel, 1990).

Health Problems

Have you ever had a bad cold and felt so miserable that all you wanted to do was go home and lie on the couch in front of the television? Eventually, you managed to get home, changed into your nightclothes and a robe, and refused to answer your telephone. The last thing you may have wanted to do is visit with friends. The same may hold true for older adults who are experiencing physical illness, physiological decline resulting from the onset of a disease, pain, fatigue, or some other sort of disability. Older adults who do not feel well may not want to be around other people. Often, low morale is associated with the onset of physical illness. As a result, some older adults actually may desire more privacy to limit interaction, to suffer alone rather than subject friends to their troubles, or to hide their illnesses from others.

Some older people may not want privacy but have trouble remaining active because of health problems. For instance, many older people experience losses in sensory capacity, such as seeing and hearing; a reduced energy level; the potential for broken bones; and chronic diseases that can have an adverse impact on mobility. (Volume 2 covers this topic in more detail.) Many older people may be forced to limit social interaction and activities as a result of these conditions. For example, it can be difficult for an older adult who is hard of hearing to carry on a conversation in a social situation. It is often impossible for him or her to discriminate between background noise and the voice of the person he or she is talking with. People who are hard of hearing also may be forced to speak louder, which can increase an older adult's concern with being overheard or becoming the subject of gossip. In addition, many older adults stop going out and socializing because they are afraid that they may not be able to find a public restroom when needed. Others may be dealing with incontinence and would be embarrassed if friends became aware of their problem.

In addition, many of these sensory losses and chronic diseases can result in the need for care assistance. Help with transferring from a wheelchair to a toilet or help with bathing can infringe on privacy. Our society places great emphasis on managing personal hygiene and bodily functions in private, and most people are accustomed to using the bathroom alone without any help. With the onset of health problems, older adults may have no choice but to involve someone else in these private situations. They may also be forced into maintaining more intimate distances from others than they might choose and may be forced to adjust to invasions of their personal space by caregivers. This subject is addressed in more detail in "What Staff Can Do" and "What the Environment Can Do" later in this chapter.

Relocation

Gino has just moved by himself from the East Coast to a new home in the Midwest to start a new job. He does not know anyone in the area and has not had a chance to join any social groups. His co-workers are friendly but rarely socialize outside of the office. Gino's family lives back east but he stays in touch via the telephone. After 2 weeks in his new home, a flood destroys a portion of the house while Gino is at work. Most of his possessions are salvaged, but it is going to take 2 or 3 weeks for the insurance claim to be filed and repairs to be made before he can live in his home again. Gino does not want to jeopardize his new job by taking time off to go back east to his family, and he certainly cannot afford to stay in a hotel for an extended period. However, his new neighbors have generously offered to put him up for a little while. Despite the kindness of his neighbors, Gino feels a little awkward about sharing a bathroom and eating meals with people he hardly knows. He realizes, however, that it is only for a short time and gratefully accepts.

What must it be like for older adults who must give up their homes and move into a long-term care facility for the rest of their lives? Many older people today live alone or with a spouse in a privately owned, single-family house. When they move into a long-term care facility, they may then find themselves eating meals with a group of unrelated strangers. They also may hear their medical situation being discussed openly at a nurse's station, or they may, for the first time in their lives, be seen in their nightclothes by many others on their way to a tub room. These changes certainly can be unsettling.

How unsettling the move is can be influenced by the policies imposed by the long-term care facility and the model of care that the facility follows.

(See Chapter 1 in this volume for additional information on the different models of care.) For example, a long-term care facility that is modeled after a hospital often emphasizes the medical needs of older people as well as schedules and care plans that promote staff convenience. As a result, staff may enter the rooms of "patients" in the morning without knocking, wake them up, and transport them by wheelchair in their nightclothes to a central bathing area. Staff may be concerned primarily with getting their residents ready in time for a 7:00 A.M. breakfast in the common dining room, and may not consider privacy needs by, for example, allowing time for residents to put on a robe. In addition, many of the bedrooms in such a long-term care facility are identical to hospital rooms—two beds are placed side by side, sometimes with a curtain drawn between them. This type of room arrangement certainly does not facilitate privacy.

Facilities that deliberately follow the hospitality model usually provide a combination of high-service hospitality and health care services in a professionally managed environment that is similar to that of a resort or hotel. In fact, staff often are trained in hospitality skills that are similar to those used in residential hotels. Residents are often treated as guests, and everything, ranging from housekeeping and laundry to personal care assistance, is done for them. Whereas some residents are receptive to this kind of help because they feel they are paying for it, others may not be prepared for the invasion of privacy that they must experience in the process.

HOW DEMENTIA AFFECTS PRIVACY

Older people with dementia experience a loss of cognitive functioning that can have an adverse impact on privacy for them as well as others who come into contact with them. Many individuals with dementia may desire more privacy, especially in the early stage, to hide their cognitive decline from family members and close friends. They may fear being in unfamiliar surroundings with unfamiliar people or misinterpreting a given situation and being viewed as foolish or hostile. They also may realize that they are exhibiting socially inappropriate behavior at times. This may cause them to withdraw because they do not know how others will react to them, or they may feel embarrassed or upset by their behavior. When others do react negatively, older adults with dementia may sense this and withdraw as a result.

As dementia progresses, older adults may exhibit disruptive behaviors if they perceive that their privacy is threatened. For example, combative behaviors toward staff often occur during assistance with dressing and bathing—acts that usually are managed in private. (See Volume 3, Chapter 5 for a discussion of combative behavior.) Because many older adults with dementia have trouble recognizing and identifying faces, places, objects, and events, they may not understand why they are being undressed, may not recognize the staff member providing assistance, and may feel embarrassed by such intimacy. They also may not be able to communicate their desire for privacy or know how to seek it or achieve it. How would you feel if someone you did not recognize was undressing you in a tub room, which may not look like a typical bathroom, with other residents and staff around?

Residents with dementia also may exhibit other types of disruptive behaviors that can have an adverse impact on the privacy of others. For instance, rummaging through other residents' belongings is a common complaint in long-term care facilities. (Rummaging is addressed in more detail in Volume 3, Chapter 4.) Residents who are cognitively intact or in the early stage of dementia often are offended by this behavior because it infringes on their privacy. Staff also may become frustrated if the nurses' station becomes the target of rummagers. With dementia, many older adults lose their sense of ownership and will pick up anything that looks interesting. If someone tries to take it away, then they may become upset and say that it is theirs. Older adults with dementia also may believe that others are stealing from them. In addition, some residents with dementia may not recognize the difference between a public and a private space and might disrobe in a public area. Again, this can be offensive to others who do not understand why certain residents are engaging in this behavior.

WHAT STAFF CAN DO

After moving into a long-term care facility, older people often desire more privacy so that they can control the information they choose to reveal as well as the amount of social interaction they desire. Staff can help protect the privacy of residents in a number of ways. Many of the recommendations provided here are directed toward administrators and refer to policies that can be implemented. Although these suggestions are directed at the administrative level, all staff should be involved, and their input should be considered. In addition, administration should determine whether the official policies actually are being practiced. It is important to track staff practices in case additional training is needed. Other recommendations are directed more toward staff directly involved in caregiving for residents. If these recommendations are implemented, then administration must fully support staff.

Develop Policies to Protect Privacy

Once a long-term care facility has decided that residents' privacy is important, several management policies should be developed based on input from all levels of staff. These policies should reflect an understanding of the importance of privacy as well as a concern for respecting a resident's personhood.

Knock Before Entering

Although most facilities have a policy that requires staff to knock on residents' bedroom doors before entry, it is often not followed, or staff may not wait for a response. Staff may feel that they do not have time to knock. They may also believe that the residents are so confused that they cannot answer or that their response does not really matter. Yet, their response *does* matter. Even if residents cannot articulate their desires verbally or staff cannot interpret what residents mean, staff still should provide residents with the opportunity to respond. Staff should not assume that residents are not always aware of events going on around them. To determine how well this policy is followed at the facility, simply observe staff as unobtrusively as possible as they go in and out of residents' rooms. Keep a count of the number of times that staff knock and wait for a reply. If the number of times that knocking does not occur is significantly greater than the number of times knocking does occur, then the facility may need to do an in-service training session on the importance of this policy. In addition, residents should have the option of keeping their bedroom doors open or closed during the day and at night. The facility should review policies and practices related to bedroom doors.

Knocking on doors at night while residents are sleeping to conduct routine night checks probably would not be appreciated. Facility policy should require staff to consult with residents and family members to determine whether residents would like this type of monitoring to continue. Some may welcome such an intrusion of privacy from a safety standpoint. Providing routine night checks for all residents whether or not they need or desire monitoring reflects a medical model of care.

Offer Help Discreetly

When providing assistance with care, staff should be taught to approach residents and ask them, in a discreet manner, if they would like help. If this conversation occurs in a public area such as a hallway or a dining room, then staff should speak directly into a resident's ear so that others nearby cannot overhear. This is an issue particularly with toileting. When parents ask young children in front of other people whether they need to go to the bathroom, it is generally considered socially acceptable. As children get older, they may roll their eyes and feel embarrassed when their parents ask about their need to go to the bathroom. Eventually, parents stop asking. Although it may be appropriate with some residents to ask or remind them to go to the bathroom, they should be treated with dignity and respect. Residents are adults and should not be treated like children.

Staff also should explain what is going to take place when offering help. Again, this should be done discreetly if you are in a public space. Because many older adults with dementia have trouble recognizing and identifying faces, places, objects, and events, they may not understand why they are being undressed or bathed, may not recognize the staff member providing assistance, and may feel embarrassed by such intimacy.

Provide Bathing Assistance in Private

In long-term care facilities, maintaining privacy can be difficult in tub rooms with multiple tubs or showers. Adequate privacy often is defined as visual separation, which has led to the use of the privacy curtain. However, these curtains do not provide acoustic or olfactory privacy. Unless each tub and shower is an enclosed, visually and acoustically private room, ideally, residents should be bathed one at a time. This can be accomplished by developing bathing schedules that eliminate the need to bathe many people at once. You may want to review your schedule of frequency of baths. How often is a full bath or shower for each resident really needed? When sponge baths are offered once or twice a week, you may be able to alleviate crowding.

If separate bathing times are not possible, then staff can use other strategies to try to make the bathing area more private. The facility can develop a policy that restricts staff from entering the area when someone is being bathed. If the tub room is being used for the storage of supplies and soiled linen carts, then consider moving the supplies and carts to another part of the facility so that staff can access these items without interrupting bathing. Music also can be used to cover up the sounds of others, and aromatherapy can mask odors. In addition, residents who are still highly concerned with privacy should not be in the tub room at the same time as residents who are normally combative during bathing.

Establish Private Spaces and Times

The facility also should develop policies for designating private times and spaces in the building. This is particularly important for residents who share bedrooms. First, the facility can schedule certain times for residents to be alone in their rooms. However, arranging this can be challenging: Roommates may not want to leave their rooms, and staff certainly cannot ask them to leave against their wishes. Second, the facility can designate at least one space for private use. This space should be both visually and acoustically private and can be used for residents who wish to spend time alone, for visits with family and friends, and for times when two residents wish to be intimate. (This topic is discussed further in Volume 3, Chapter 6. Suggestions for ways to create private spaces are included in "What the Environment Can Do" later in this chapter.) Such efforts to provide private spaces and times are important because research has shown that increased opportunities for privacy lead to greater levels of social interaction throughout the facility (Calkins, 1991).

Recognize Residents' Privacy Needs

The following discussion focuses on ways that staff, particularly direct care staff, can play a vital role in implementing policies that protect the privacy of residents.

Gather Information About the Resident's History

Staff should gather information about each resident's personal history as it relates to issues of privacy. Staff can gather such information by meeting with residents and family members and asking them about a resident's privacy needs. Some of the questions should concern the resident's past behavior. Did the resident spend great amounts of time alone before moving into the long-term care facility? Did he or she live alone? Was the resident social? Are there certain things the resident does not like to discuss? Some residents may be sensitive to certain experiences, such as serving in World War II, and staff should not bring up such an issue in conversation. Are there certain activities, such as doing crossword puzzles or watching television, that the resident liked to pursue when alone?

Staff then should determine whether the facility is supporting the privacy needs of the resident. Are appropriate supplies and props available in the facility to engage a resident in activities that he or she likes to pursue alone? Are there opportunities for social interaction? Is the resident forced to participate in social activities even though he or she is a loner? In addition, staff should observe residents in the facility to try to gain an understanding of their current privacy needs, because dementia may have altered their previous behavior patterns. A Resident Social History form and a Previous Housing Experience form are included in Appendix A of this volume. These forms can assist staff with the collection of pertinent information on each resident.

Redirect Residents Infringing on the Privacy of Others

Certain behaviors, such as rummaging and hoarding, can infringe on the privacy of others living in long-term care facilities. Residents who are cognitively intact often are offended when other residents go through their belongings and do not listen to their requests to leave them and their possessions alone. This issue may be one of orientation: Residents may be rummaging because they are confused by the possessions in another resident's room. Several interventions may help to redirect residents. Places to rummage can be created; residents can be encouraged to be productive by, for example, collecting items based on a theme; and sensory stimulation can be increased through activities, tactile art, and miscellaneous objects that are accessible and easy to pick up and hold. (Volume 3, Chapter 4 covers these and other suggestions in more detail.) In addition, volunteers may be able to take someone off the unit if staff do not have time to redirect residents.

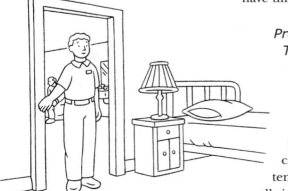

Provide Bathing and Toileting Assistance in Private

Our society places great emphasis on managing personal hygiene and bodily functions in private. Staff who provide care assistance for residents often find themselves in a personally intimate situation that demands close proximity. To deal with what can be an uncomfortable situation, staff may try to distance themselves by body posture and minimal eye contact. This can suggest that staff also are distancing themselves from the resident as a person. By providing privacy for residents during personal care assistance, both residents and staff may benefit.

Privacy can be provided in a variety of ways. For example, in facilities with tub rooms, residents should have the option of undressing in the tub room or in their bedrooms. If residents choose to undress in their bedrooms, then staff should avoid draping them in a towel or a sheet when helping them down the hallway to the tub room. A robe owned by the resident would be more appropriate. During bathing, staff should consider covering residents with a sheet and washing their bodies under the sheet. This type of bathing protects the privacy of residents who are concerned about being nude in front of "strangers," and also helps to minimize disruptive behaviors such as combativeness. Often, these behaviors occur when older adults perceive that their privacy is threatened.

In addition, staff should respect the privacy of residents who need assistance with toileting. For residents who just need to be taken to the bathroom and possibly helped onto the toilet, staff may be able to step outside the bathroom while residents are voiding. When residents let staff know that they are finished, staff can return and provide any additional assistance that is needed. For people who need step-by-step cueing once inside the bathroom, staff may be able to turn their backs while the resident is voiding or having a bowel movement.

WHAT THE ENVIRONMENT CAN DO

Many possibilities exist for increasing opportunities for privacy in long-term care settings through alteration of physical features. Changes to both the inside and outside of buildings can help to provide privacy. This discussion starts with the more private areas of the facility by first looking at shared resident bedrooms and bathrooms. It then addresses hallways and indoor and outdoor shared spaces such as living rooms, lobbies, tub rooms, outdoor courtyards, and garden areas.

Shared Residents' Bedrooms

Many people often ask, what is the right proportion of private versus shared bedrooms in a long-term care facility? No available research can answer that question. Nevertheless, anecdotal information suggests that private rooms usually are preferred. In general, a facility should have one shared bedroom for every 6–12 private bedrooms. Privacy can be difficult to achieve in shared bedrooms. Yet, just as in a house, the bedroom is the most private area of a long-term care setting. Certain furniture arrangements and room assignments can help enhance privacy in shared bedrooms without radically altering the bedroom arrangement.

Furniture Arrangements

In shared bedrooms in long-term care facilities, two beds often are placed side by side, with a privacy curtain between them. Usually, this does not meet residents' privacy needs. Other options that should be considered include building display cases, bookcases, or solid, half-height partition walls with a display shelf on top between the beds. At the very least, such an arrangement provides a clearer sense of personal space and opportunities for personalization. However, one person will still "own" the window; the other person will be forced to deal with people invading his or her space to enter and exit the bedroom; and acoustic, olfactory, and thermal privacy will not be enhanced. Where space permits, beds can also be placed toe-to-toe with a solid partition between the beds. Rooms may feel more private as a result. For administrators who are contemplating major renovations or new construction, an L-shaped arrangement in which each bed is in a separate alcove is another option (see Figure 4.1).

Room Assignments

The facility may want to assign residents to private or semiprivate bedrooms based on the location of the rooms and the privacy needs of residents. For example, certain bedrooms are located in parts of the facility that are noisier than other parts. They may be near a nurse's station, a dining room, or a living room. Residents who have a greater tolerance for noise or who like to be where the action is should be placed in these bedrooms. In contrast, residents who desire greater privacy should be placed in bedrooms that are toward the far ends of hallways. However, bedrooms that are directly at the ends of hallways are more likely to be entered accidentally by residents who are wanderers. Residents who are less concerned with privacy, have a higher tolerance for intrusions, and welcome interaction should be placed in those rooms. At the same time, the facility should provide a locked and secure storage space in each bedroom for possessions about which residents may be concerned. This is advisable for private bedrooms as well.

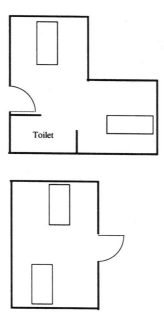

Figure 4.1. Beds can be placed in an L-shaped or toe-to-toe configuration to enhance privacy in a shared bedroom.

Residents' Bathrooms

Privacy is an important issue in resident bathrooms. The facility may have to balance the importance of privacy with the need to provide orientation cues to help residents independently maintain continence. (Orientation is covered in more detail in Volume 2, Chapter 2). For example, toilets that are highly visible often help to reduce incontinence. If incontinence is a problem in the facility, then consider removing doors to bathrooms and replacing them with privacy curtains.

Hallways

Where hallways are wider than the required minimum width imposed by state regulations, opportunities for varying degrees of privacy and social interaction can be provided by establishing small seating areas along hallways outside the flow of traffic (Figure 4.2). Residents can stop to rest or people-watch in these areas.

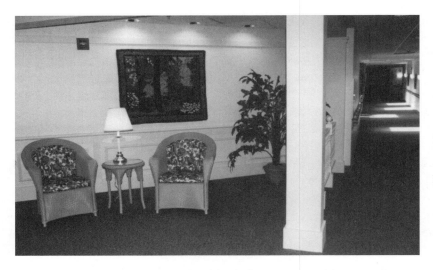

Figure 4.2.   Small seating areas in wider hallways can provide spaces for residents to control privacy and social interaction.

Nooks along hallways that are outside shared spaces such as living rooms also can provide opportunities for residents to spend time by themselves or to watch ongoing activities without having to participate. Bedroom doorways that are recessed and grouped together can provide residents with opportunities for more private contact with neighbors.

Indoor Shared Spaces

Opportunities for residents to control privacy and social interaction are also advantageous in shared indoor spaces, including living rooms, lobbies, and activity rooms. People do not live only in their bedrooms, and strategies that enhance privacy should be devised to encourage the use of these spaces. Seating arrangements and the division of large spaces into smaller, less overwhelming ones can help.

Seating Arrangements

Several different types of furniture arrangements should be provided in indoor spaces to encourage some residents to engage in group activities while allowing others the opportunity to be alone or watch the residents who are engaged in activities. A proper balance is vital. When chairs are arranged in small clusters at right angles to one another, for example, people are more likely to interact because this furniture grouping facilitates communication.

The same is true for chairs arranged around small tables. Gaps between chairs in small clusters or around tables may encourage residents with assistive devices to join the group. In contrast, chairs lined up around the perimeter of a room are not particularly welcoming. For those individuals who wish only to look rather than participate or interact, a single chair overlooking a window or a chair with its back to other furniture provides more privacy.

Division of Space

Dividing large rooms into smaller, less overwhelming spaces can decrease confusion and agitation and provide opportunities for balancing privacy and social interaction. This can be accomplished with furniture and folding partition walls (see the "Where to Find Products" section for sources for dividers). These allow flexibility because spaces can be divided and opened up depending on the activity that is taking place. A more permanent solution is the provision of half-walls, possibly with glass above them. This differentiates space and allows some visibility between areas. This type of division is desirable for residents who wish to view activities before making a commitment to participate or socialize. If the glass in the upper half of the walls is equipped with blinds or shades, then visual separation between spaces can be provided when necessary. (See Figure 4.3 for examples of divider configurations in dining rooms.)

When dividing up a larger room, it is also important to recognize that certain parts of that space are more secluded when they are not directly visible from a nurse's station, a hallway, or an entry. You may want to develop this part of the room as a more private space for individual activities. In contrast, highly visible spaces may be appropriate for activities that are meant to attract more people and encourage participation.

Tub Rooms

If separate bathing times are not possible in tub rooms, then strategies can be used to try to make the bathing areas more private. For example, supply and soiled linen carts should be located in another part of the facility so that staff do not have to access these items when residents are bathing. Music can be used to cover up the sounds of other residents, and aromatherapy can hide odors. Half-height shower curtains that provide some privacy for residents when sitting and keep caregivers dry are useful as well. (See "Where to Find Products" for sources of aromatherapy products and half-height curtains.) Walls can be built to increase separation between different bathing areas if this is economically feasible. In addition, hooks for robes, clothes, and personal towels should be provided so that residents can undress and dress in the tub room rather than having to wait until they get back to their rooms.

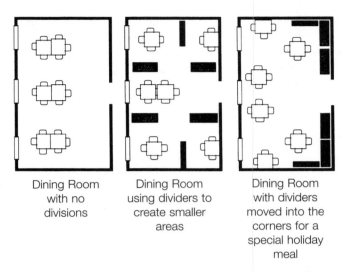

| Dining Room with no divisions | Dining Room using dividers to create smaller areas | Dining Room with dividers moved into the corners for a special holiday meal |

Figure 4.3. Examples of divider configurations in dining rooms.

Outdoor Shared Spaces

As with interior shared spaces, opportunities for people to control privacy and social interaction are important in outdoor shared spaces such as courtyards, patios, and garden areas. Principles regarding seating arrangements and the division of indoor space, as discussed previously, apply to outdoor areas as well. Outside, however, spaces can be divided into smaller areas with outdoor furniture, including tables and chairs and porch swings, garden planters, retaining walls, and landscaping. Within these spaces, the facility should provide opportunities for individual activities such as sitting in the sun or bird watching, as well as activities that involve group interaction. In addition, views of and access to an enclosed outdoor area can increase residents' options in seeking out privacy or social interaction.

WHERE TO FIND PRODUCTS

Cabinets for Dividing Dining Rooms

Adden Furniture, Inc.
26 Jackson Street
Lowell, MA 01852
(508) 457-7848

Allsteel, Inc.
Allsteel Drive
Aurora, IL 60507
(800) 764-2535
www.allsteeloffice.com
Allsteel's InterChange panel system consists of dividers with acoustical inserts on both sides. The company also offers a variety of wheeled cabinets for storage.

Aromatherapy

Gaiam
(formerly Selfcare)
360 Interlocken Boulevard, Suite 300
Broomfield, CO 80021-3440
(877) 989-6321
www.gaiam.com

Half-Height Shower Curtains

Invacare
528 Hughes Drive
Traverse City, MI 49683
(800) 678-7100
www.invacare-ccg.com
Invacare manufactures a low shower curtain that provides privacy and protects those giving the bath.

◆ ◆ ◆

A summary sheet follows, which condenses the chapter text into a quick overview. The authors have also provided an area for you to make your own notes about your own staff and facility. Managerial staff may wish to use the summary sheets as handouts to accompany direct care staff training, or to post them by the time clock or nurses' station or include them in staff's pay envelopes.

PRIVACY SUMMARY SHEET

1. Privacy is the ability to control who you see, when you see others, and what information others have or know about you.
2. You do not truly have privacy if someone can walk in on you unannounced or unexpectedly.
3. When you are in private, you can really "let your hair down" and be yourself.
4. Older adults experience major changes (losses) in privacy between living at home and living in a shared residential setting.

What Staff Can Do

1. Knock on doors before entering *at all times.* Wait for an answer, or open the door a little and wave to signal that you are coming in.
2. Determine whether routine night checks are really medically necessary for care or are desired by each resident.
3. Find ways to minimize the extent during dressing and bathing to which residents are naked in front of others by draping a sheet or only partially undressing one part of the body at a time.
4. Establish times for privacy, especially for residents who share rooms.
5. Do not talk about a resident's condition, medical needs, or care plans in public areas where you could be overheard.
6. Be discrete when helping a resident to the toilet.

What the Environment Can Do

1. Use room dividers to create small, private areas.
2. Never bathe more than one resident at a time in the same tub room.

YOUR NOTES

5

Autonomy and Control

Maria was awakened by her alarm clock this morning. She was not too happy when the buzzer sounded, but she was able to find the clock—right where she positioned it the night before—to hit the snooze button. Maria had decided to set her alarm just a little bit earlier so that she could hit the snooze button a couple of times before having to get up for work. When getting out of bed, she found her bedroom cold and decided to turn up the thermostat. Because Maria had hit the 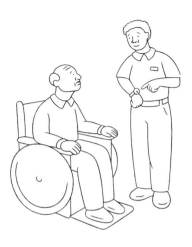 *snooze button on her clock so many times, she decided that a shower would be quicker than a bath. Then, she opted to have cereal for breakfast rather than scrambled eggs and toast. Maria chose to eat in the living room so that she could watch the morning news on television.*

The activities mentioned in the example are often taken for granted, yet they are important for many reasons. We are able to find our clocks when the alarm sounds because we have decorated and arranged our bedrooms and are familiar with them as a result. We are free to adjust the thermostat, without consulting others, because we feel cold. We also have the opportunity to choose between getting up right away or snoozing a little longer, as well as taking a shower or a bath, and to decide what to have for breakfast. We are aware of the consequences of all of these decisions. Furthermore, we are able to follow these routines in an order that we established and personally find comfortable and predictable. In all cases, we have influence over our behavior or actions, our time, our thinking and decision making, and our environment. These are factors that contribute to autonomy or control (Edney, 1975).

Our society places great emphasis on control. Deciding when to get up and what to eat for breakfast, for example, is a part of the right to control our lives, a right that we expect to possess as law-abiding, competent adults. However, we give certain individuals or groups the power to take away such rights to self-determination. The legal system can place criminals in jail and deny them many of their rights. Parents often restrict the rights of children until they are mature enough to make competent decisions and act accordingly. Adult children sometimes restrict the autonomy of aging parents by placing them in a long-term care facility against their will. The right to control also varies depending on the circumstances or setting in which we find ourselves. For example, office environments typically impose certain rules. You usually have to be at work by a certain time and may have to follow a dress code. Similarly, you may have to dress up to go to church or temple or out to dinner at a fancy restaurant.

It is in the personal territory of your home that you, as a mature, competent adult, usually can act as you wish, make decisions as you like, and structure your time to suit your personal desires. Control is important to all people because people like to exercise choice and to have influence over their decisions and actions. This usually leads to feelings of well-being.

CHOICE

As you searched for your current home, you probably had a choice between different neighborhoods and various homes. The taxes in certain neighborhoods and the prices and maintenance costs of certain houses or apartments may have limited your options, but you still had some choice. Once you moved in, you were also able to choose where you would like to shop, where to attend religious services, and where you would like to get your car fixed. These are important because "people have the capacity to make choices and the desire to exercise this capacity" (Cantril, 1978, p. 97). Of course, choice requires that some options exist. If there were only one grocery store or car repair shop within 20 miles of your home, then you would not really have much of a choice.

Having too many choices can be overwhelming. Have you ever been in a restaurant where the menu is just too long? You may have found it difficult to read through the entire menu, to remember all of the choices, and to decide among the many dishes that you found appealing. In contrast, too few choices can result in boredom. For example, there may be only one place to eat near your office and it has a limited lunch menu. After a few weeks, you may grow tired of eating the same two or three dishes for lunch. In addition, your choices must be meaningful, must be consistent with your preferences and values, and must allow you to express your individuality. For vegetarians, for example, having the choice of a turkey sandwich or a hamburger for lunch would be useless.

WELL-BEING

How would you feel if intruders broke into your house and tied your wrists and ankles together before taking your possessions? Imagine if you were left that way after the intruders escaped. While waiting for someone to discover your plight, you were not free to move and could not leave your home. Aside from feeling violated and frightened as a result of the robbery, you would probably feel as if you have no control. Prisoners of war and people in concentration camps as well as patients in mental hospitals in the early part of the twentieth century probably felt many of the same feelings you would have experienced as a victim of robbery. However, probably you would come to the realization soon that someone will miss you, and eventually you will be discovered. In contrast, prisoners, people in concentration camps, and psychiatric patients often did not foresee a change in their situation. Many suffered apathy and withdrawal as a result of feeling helpless to control their lives. Research has indicated that learned helplessness develops when people repeatedly are exposed to uncontrollable events and, as a result, believe that their individual actions cannot influence future outcomes (Seligman, 1975, cited in Pinet, 1985).

When people are able to make their own decisions, act on them, and retain a sense of control over their lives in the process, they usually feel good about themselves. Alternatively, this is a right that we, as a society, take away from those who violate our laws, by putting them in prison, which severely reduces their ability to make decisions, and exercise control and autonomy. For example, you would probably experience satisfaction and peace of mind if you were able to accept an invitation to a party, dress as you pleased, drive to the party, eat and drink what you want, talk with whomever you find interesting, and leave when you are ready. This sense of control can certainly lead to feelings of well-being.

Feelings of well-being, however, can result from actual control or perceived control. Perceived control refers to the belief that people have the ability to control their environment and are not influenced by outside forces. This is different from actual control or the ability to implement control. For example, your teenage child may want to go out with his or her friends to catch a late movie in town. As a parent, you are concerned and may tell your child that he or she can meet these friends at an earlier showing of the movie or invite them back to the house to watch a rented movie. In this sense, you are allowing your child to exert some control, which may lead the child to believe that he or she is in control and is making a choice. In actuality, you are tailoring his or her options.

Feelings of well-being are also related to people's desire for control. How much autonomy people desire can vary depending on different life experiences. For instance, those who have adapted to living with many people because they were raised in a large family might have less of a need to exercise control. For many American families, particularly older generations, women controlled certain areas of the home, such as the kitchen, while men were responsible for areas outside of the house, such as the yard and garage. With retirement, however, many men try to take over parts of the house that women traditionally have controlled, which can lead to conflict. Different personalities can affect people's desire for control as well. For example, people referred to as having a "type A personality" usually exhibit competitive traits, have a great need to achieve, and act with a great sense of urgency. Research has shown that individuals with this personality type often cope with uncontrollable stress by actively trying to seek out and assert as much control over a situation as possible (Glass, 1977, cited in Pinet, 1985).

In contrast, feelings of well-being can be related to having less control. Individuals who exhibit the pattern of behavior of a "type B personality" may feel stressed if they have a high degree of control over a situation. All people do not want the same amount of control. Some people, for instance, actually prefer to have some decisions made for them, possibly because having control can imply responsibility. The potential effort that is associated with responsibility can lead to dissatisfaction (Gifford, 1997). In other words, some people care more about "things being under control" than about "having control" (Kaplan, 1983). Other people may prefer less control because they derive satisfaction from predictability rather than control. "The ability to reliably predict when, where, and for how long positive or negative events are likely to happen is almost as beneficial as actual control over these occurrences" (Calkins, 1988, p. 15). For instance, even though you do not have control over the fact that you must show up to work every day at 7:00 A.M., there may be some benefits associated with your routine schedule. Imagine how confusing it would be if your shift started at a different time each day.

HOW AUTONOMY AND CONTROL CHANGE WITH AGE AND RELOCATION

Throughout life, the need for control or autonomy remains important. Even as people age, they still need to have control or be in control to exercise choice and to enhance feelings of well-being. This may become an even greater need in the later stages of life when older adults experience many significant social and health-related losses. When older adults must move into a long-term care facility, however, they may end up with fewer opportunities to exercise control. This can affect their sense of well-being negatively (Figure 5.1).

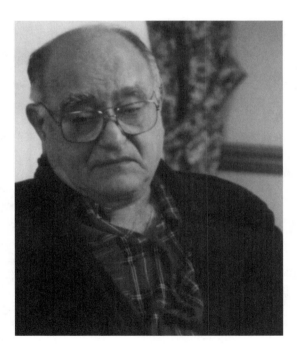

Figure 5.1. Older adults have fewer opportunities to exercise control in long-term care facilities, which can result in helplessness, depression, and physical decline.

Social and Physical Losses

Harry's boss informed him one day that it was time for Harry to think about retiring. Harry still took pride in his work, received a certain amount of satisfaction, and really did not want to retire. His unsympathetic boss told Harry that he would enjoy all of his new free time. For a moment, Harry thought that retirement might not be too bad. He could do all of the things he had been putting off for years. For instance, he had always wanted to improve his golf game. But then Harry realized that he was going to have to deal with a reduction in income after retiring. He might not have the money he would need for golf. All of a sudden, free time really did not seem appealing.

For many older adults, retirement from paid work can result in the loss of a role that may have been a significant source of control. This can be compounded when older adults are forced into retirement or must manage their lives on a reduced income. Similarly, the child-rearing role may have been a meaningful source of control. As children grow up and move away, however, older adults must gradually come to terms with giving up control (see Chapter 3 for additional information on role loss). For example, many older adults may have always had Christmas dinner at their homes. As they age, they may find that it is too much effort to cook for so many people and may be forced to hand over the tradition to their children. Older adults also may have to deal with the psychological loss of control as more and more loved ones from their cohort pass on, and the next generation takes over.

Perhaps the greatest loss of control for older adults is associated with sensory changes and physical decline. (Volume 2 covers this topic in much more detail.) A loss in sensory capacities such as vision and hearing, a reduced energy level, and chronic conditions, such as high blood pressure, arthritis, and heart disease all can have an adverse impact on an individual. These changes can limit activities, interaction, and self-care abilities and can give older people a feeling that they are losing control of their bodies. Impaired vision, hearing, and speech can prevent older people from communicating their wishes if they need assistance. This can be compounded by the humiliation and embarrassment that many older adults may feel at not being able to execute simple procedures such as tying their shoes or by the need to wear incontinence pads. This may lead to a heightened need to exercise control. A loss of control can also result in depression, helplessness (Schulz, 1976, cited in Calkins, 1988), an unwillingness to cooperate with medical treatments that require physical effort, greater recovery time from illness, and additional physical decline (Rodin, 1986).

Relocation

Someone entered Edna's bedroom this morning without knocking and woke her out of a deep sleep by opening the curtains and letting the sun stream in. She could not recognize the person because she did not have her glasses on and they were not on the night table where she left them the night before. The person who entered Edna's room then told her that it was her turn for a shower but that she would have to hurry because the person was already behind schedule. The person then started rummaging through her closet and picked out something for her to wear. Edna asked for her glasses, but the person said there was no time left to look for them.

Events such as these are typical of what many older adults must cope with after moving into a long-term care facility. These events may happen for many reasons. First, the older person's routine way of doing things may not work in the new living arrangement. Rooms are arranged differently and may not include familiar possessions from residents' previous homes. In addition, some spaces are shared with other residents. Many older adults may have grown accustomed to living alone and controlling their home environment once children moved away, a spouse died, or both. In a long-term care facility, however, residents must live in close proximity with many unrelated strangers and come to terms with shared control. Rights and preferences of many individuals as well as the rights of the group as a whole must be considered. As a result, older residents may feel as if they cannot control things such as lighting in shared spaces or the amount of social contact they must cope with in hallways daily.

Second, personal autonomy in a long-term care facility is often sacrificed because of concerns for safety, risk, and sanitation. Protecting residents from physical harm is usually a priority among health care providers. Building codes, federal and state regulations, and care practices are usually designed to ensure physical safety for residents. For example, a resident may be discouraged from skipping a meal even if he or she was used to eating only two meals a day—a late breakfast and a main meal in the early evening—as a result of nutritional requirements imposed by federal regulations. Staff may provide more assistance with a shower than is necessary for fear that a resident may slip, fall, and break a bone. This care practice may be applied across the board to all residents regardless of individual physical and cognitive abilities. Constant surveillance by staff can result. A fear of liability may cause the facility to resist experimenting with alternative practices that might involve reasonable risks but enhance the residents' sense of control.

Third, the model of care the facility follows can have an impact on personal autonomy (see Chapter 1 in this volume for additional information on models of care). A facility that embraces the medical model often views aging as a medical problem and residents as patients rather than as people with individual psychosocial needs. This can establish a relationship in which caregivers tell residents what to do, and residents are expected to follow doctors' orders. Residents who do not cooperate are considered difficult. Besides actual medical care, the people with whom residents eat, when they eat, what they eat, and what they wear may be decided by staff for the residents' own good. Facilities that follow the medical model usually are driven by rigid schedules and task-oriented routines. Residents may be told, for example, that they do not have a choice between a shower and a bath. They may be given one or the other depending on which is most convenient and efficient for staff. Such regimentation can contribute to a loss of control. In addition, the medical model emphasizes medical care that is reimbursable. "Everything becomes 'therapy' so that it qualifies for reimbursement. Music therapy, activity therapy, and pet therapy are attempts to make psychosocial needs of clients conform to the medical model" (Hofland & David, 1990, p. 93). A facility that follows a hospitality model of care may restrict choices and control as well. In this case, staff usually do everything for residents, much in the same way that a hotel caters to its guests, because residents are paying for this service. However, some residents may not like this lifestyle.

Fourth, staff may not view residents as their clients. Family members may have helped residents relocate or may have placed them in a long-term care facility against their will. Family members also may be the ones paying the bills and often are most vocal about concerns over care practices. As a result, staff frequently consult with families rather than residents when making caregiving decisions. Yet it is not always clear that family members are acting in the best interest of residents or effectively voicing concerns residents may have (Walsh, 1990). This may be because family members may not be aware that their wishes differ from the needs of the older person with dementia. In addition, many older adults of this cohort were raised in an era when assertiveness was discouraged and considered impolite (Walsh, 1990). Challenging family members or authority figures such as care providers may not be something many older people feel comfortable doing.

HOW DEMENTIA AFFECTS AUTONOMY AND CONTROL

The move to a long-term care facility and the accompanying loss of control certainly can be a traumatic experience for older people. It can be especially traumatic for older people with dementia. They may feel not only as if they are losing control of their bodies as a result of health-related losses and their social lives because of the death of loved ones but also as if they are losing their minds as a result of dementia. To make matters worse, moving from the familiar surroundings and routines of a previous home to an unfamiliar long-term care setting often intensifies the confused states of people with dementia.

In the early stage of dementia, older adults usually are aware of their cognitive losses. As a result, they may realize that they literally are losing their minds. How would you feel if you could not remember what you had for breakfast this morning, could not remember your children's names, or could not remember how to get to work? How would you feel if this were something you were aware of and could not change? You would probably feel frustrated, frightened, and out of control. You might feel a need to try to exert even more control over your environment. This may be exhibited, however, by rummaging through drawers or closets in an effort to find something that looks familiar and comforting, although that can be upsetting to others or infringe on others' sense of control.

In the later stages of dementia, older adults may be less concerned with control. As a result of memory deficits and aphasia, they may be less able to communicate their wishes. Caregivers also may take more and more control away from residents with dementia for safety and security reasons. Yet we do not really know how people with dementia think and feel and whether we are creating excess disability by totally removing control from their lives. There is some indication that people with dementia should continue to have the opportunity to make decisions and take responsibility for their lives to the greatest extent possible (Coons & Spencer, 1983). Even if the sphere of control of people with dementia is limited to what they can see and touch, they should still have the opportunity to exercise some control. There is also some indication that older people with dementia can retain skills such as selecting clothes if they continue to engage in these activities.

WHAT STAFF CAN DO

Staff can help increase opportunities for autonomy and control for residents living in long-term care settings in a number of ways. The following discussion provides some recommendations. A number of these recommendations are directed toward administrators and refer to policies that can be implemented to encourage control. Although these suggestions are directed at the administrative level, all staff should be involved, and their input should be considered. Other recommendations are directed more toward direct care staff, including assistance with activities of daily living (ADLs). In this case, administration must fully support staff if these recommendations are implemented.

Many of the suggestions may require the facility to alter its thinking about what contributes to a sense of home. In particular, the facility may have to decide whether it really wishes to encourage residents to have more control over such things as routines, decisions about care, and the decoration of private rooms and shared spaces in the facility. This is something that all levels of staff at the facility will need to discuss in conjunction with the model of care the facility follows (unless this is dictated by a corporate/administrative entity).

Developing Policies to Encourage Control

Once a long-term care facility has decided that the residents' feeling of control is an important component of creating a sense of home in the facility, several management policies should be developed based on input from all levels of staff. These policies should reflect an understanding of the importance of control as well as a concern for respecting each individual's personhood. Sample policy topics include knocking on doors, giving residents a chance to say no, involving residents in the roommate pairing process, and developing a residents' council.

Knock Before Entering

A policy should be established that requires staff to knock on residents' bedroom doors. Whether doors are open or closed, staff should be directed to wait for a response before entering residents' bedrooms to help with ADLs. Even if residents cannot articulate their desires verbally or staff cannot interpret what residents mean, staff still should provide residents with the opportunity to respond. Staff should not assume that residents are not aware of events going on around them.

Many facilities have such a policy, but it is not always enforced, and therefore not followed. Consider unobtrusively watching staff on all shifts to document the extent to which they knock and wait for a response. If this does not happen regularly, then the facility should discuss the importance of this policy at an in-service training session or staff meeting. To convey the importance of the policy, you might think about ways to set up an invasion of staff members' privacy. For instance, ask staff how they would feel if someone walked into their house or bedroom without knocking and waiting to be invited to enter. Walk into their offices without knocking. These "real" experiences should give staff a greater understanding of what it feels like to have their privacy invaded and should help to make the point more effectively than simply telling staff to knock first.

Allow Residents to Alter Their Environment

The facility should develop policies that permit residents to alter their environment in bedrooms and private bathrooms to satisfy visual, acoustic, and thermal comfort as well as decorating tastes. For example, residents should have the option of regulating heating and air conditioning in bedrooms with individual thermostats. If individual thermostats do not exist, or residents do not know how to operate these devices, then residents should still be consulted about how warm or cool they would like to keep their bedrooms. It is important for staff to realize that residents are often colder than are staff. Consequently, an environment that is comfortable for a resident may seem overly warm to staff.

Residents also should be permitted to open windows for natural ventilation. Screens on windows should be used to keep out insects and to prevent residents from climbing out windows. Hardware stores also sell simple window locks (usually marketed for security from burglars) that limit how far a window can be opened. With some of these products, the vertical distance can be changed with a key. You should check with the local fire marshal and the facility's licensing agency for any codes that might restrict window operations. In a similar manner, residents should be able to regulate natural and artificial lighting levels by opening or closing their blinds or curtains and turning lights up or down.

Personalization of bedrooms should be strongly encouraged as well (see Chapter 2 in this volume). Residents should have the opportunity to change wall colors and floor coverings (at the occupants' expense unless the facility is planning to repaint or the resident is first taking occupancy); to add personal possessions, furniture, and window coverings; to hang artwork; and to arrange furniture to suit individual tastes. Personalization of interior and outdoor shared spaces such as living rooms, dining rooms, and garden areas also may help to give residents a greater sense of control over the entire facility. Often, a facility must work with the family at the time of admission to help them to understand the importance of having personal belongings in bedrooms and shared spaces.

Give Residents a Chance to Say No

Staff should be strongly encouraged to take residents' preferences into account. At each meal, for example, staff should ask whether residents would like salt or pepper on their food. Staff should not simply add salt or pepper or assume that this is a trivial concern. Even if residents cannot articulate their desires verbally or staff cannot interpret what residents mean, staff should still provide residents with the opportunity to accept or refuse what is being offered.

Staff should not assume that residents are unaware of events going on around them and cannot make these personal decisions.

Encourage Contact with Others

A study that addressed issues of autonomy for nursing facility residents who were cognitively intact (Kane & Freeman, n.d., documented in Walsh, 1990) found that residents would like more control over the use of the telephone as well as visiting policies. Ideally, residents should have their own telephones. If individual telephone lines in bedrooms do not exist or there is a concern about residents with dementia making unnecessary telephone calls or using other people's telephones, the facility should set aside an area where residents can make calls in private whenever they wish. Assistance can be provided if necessary, and residents can be billed for each call. In addition, the facility should consider less restrictive visiting hours. Just as you can welcome visitors into your home at any hour of the day, a policy should be developed that permits residents to visit with family and friends freely at reasonable hours. In addition, families should be encouraged to become involved in activities at the facility.

The Eden Alternative (Thomas, 1996) stresses that pets, plants, and children should be incorporated within the daily life of a facility. Residents should be encouraged to participate in the daily care of animals and plants and to develop one-to-one relationships with children. These meaningful activities can promote growth among residents and provide them with a sense of control over something in their lives. Consequently, the facility should consider policies that encourage gardening, welcome regular visits from children in the community, and permit pets in certain areas of the facility. At the same time, the facility should respect the wishes of residents who are not interested in gardening, visiting with children, or taking care of pets by not forcing them to participate in such activities despite their therapeutic benefit. These preferences should be noted on residents' charts.

Involve Residents in the Roommate Pairing Process

Many older adults have been used to living alone in a single-family house, especially after children moved away or following the death of a spouse. Sharing a space such as a bedroom and bathroom that is much smaller than the house that most have identified with over a lifetime can be traumatic. Sharing that space with an unrelated stranger can be even more traumatic. Residents, along with family members, should have the chance to participate in the roommate pairing process if private rooms are not available. Although choices may be limited when first entering the facility, residents should have the option, to the greatest extent possible, of moving in with another resident they befriend as rooms become available. In addition, preferences for certain types of roommates should be considered. For example, some residents actually prefer sharing a room with a resident who is not particularly mobile. They do not have to be concerned about being startled by a roommate coming and going and can feel a greater sense of control over the bedroom as a result.

Develop a Residents' Council

For residents who are in the early stage of dementia, a residents' council may help to incorporate resident concerns and preferences into the daily life of the facility (Kane & Freeman, n.d., documented in Walsh, 1990). Residents can meet regularly, discuss concerns they have, and present these concerns to administration for consideration. When the administration is receptive to the council and addresses reasonable concerns as needed, residents may feel that they have a greater say in their life within the facility. For others in the later stages of dementia, a family council or an ombudsman can convey resident wishes.

Providing Meaningful Choices

Staff, particularly those involved in caregiving, can play a vital role in enhancing residents' sense of control by taking into account residents' preferences that are consistent with the identity and decisional history of each individual. This is important because all residents are different, and staff often have different views on what aspects of daily life are important for residents to control in a long-term care facility (Kane, Freeman, Caplan, Aroskar, & Urv-Wong, 1990). This can be achieved by providing a range of choices with respect to assistance with ADLs as well as choices of general activities. In all cases, the intent should be to convey to residents that their needs, abilities, and preferences are important despite the fact that their bodies and minds may be deteriorating.

Consider Residents' Preferences When Providing Assistance

Residents should be provided with choices when receiving assistance with ADLs. For example, they should be provided with the option of a bath or a shower, allowed to go to bed and get up when they please, and permitted to wear what they wish. Most people have developed routines for when and how they bathe, dress, and eat meals. Upsetting this routine may cause some residents to exhibit disruptive behaviors. As a result, it is important to identify and follow as many of these routines and preferences as possible. At the same time, staff must realize that some residents may not view autonomy as beneficial. Passive individuals may prefer to be dependent on caregivers.

There are times when residents, especially those with late-stage dementia, will not be able to articulate their preferences and make choices. In such instances, family members should be consulted about residents' preferences and previous patterns of behavior. In addition, staff sometimes can determine preferences by using a behavior tracking process. If a resident is combative during showering, for example, then staff can record some basic information each time the behavior occurs to understand the cause of the behavior. Staff should record the 5 Ws—who, what (e.g., what behavior), where, when, and why. Although a number of factors may be causing the combative behavior, it may be occurring simply because the resident with dementia was used to taking baths and prefers this form of bathing to showers. (Volume 3, Chapter 1 provides more detail on the 5 Ws and the behavior tracking process, and a Behavior Tracking Form is provided in Appendix A of that volume.)

Staff can employ other simple ways to understand residents' preferences so that they can provide desirable choices. For example, food-tasting activities can be implemented. Residents can be asked to rate samples of foods or staff can observe which foods residents seem to like. The preferred foods can then be incorporated in the menu cycle (Walsh, 1990; Zgola & Bordillon, 2001) and can provide a more pleasurable eating experience. Getting dressed is another area in which staff need to be sensitive to residents' needs and abilities. Staff may dress residents who do not seem to be able to dress themselves, when in fact the problem may not be in getting dressed but in making decisions about what to wear. Rather than simply taking over all parts of dressing, staff should start by offering residents two outfits between which they can choose. Often this is all the help that residents need. If residents still require more assistance, then they should, at the very least, still have the option of choosing what to wear to feel that they are still involved in the task of dressing, can select an outfit with which they are comfortable, and have some sense of control. This is easier to accomplish when caregivers are consistently assigned to the same residents.

Once information has been collected about residents' preferences, the facility must decide what can be done to take these preferences into account and to allow routines to continue. For instance, the facility can consider how necessary it is for residents to have breakfast together or to eat breakfast at all. If state and federal regulations mandate a minimum and maximum number of hours required between meals, then a heavy snack can be served late at night to residents who prefer to sleep later than when breakfast is normally served. A continental breakfast could be offered to residents once they awaken. Staff can check with each resident's physician to determine how important breakfast is for that resident and whether an order could be written permitting a resident to skip breakfast if he or she prefers to sleep instead. In addition, information about each resident's preferences should be disseminated to all staff. Staff should be provided with the necessary time to review each resident's history.

Provide a Choice of Activities

Residents also should be provided with choices in their activities. For example, multiple activities should be scheduled simultaneously. Different kinds of activities should be offered as well, and it is important to have the various activities be *meaningfully* different. To offer a choice between coloring a picture of a girl on a beach or a boy playing baseball is not meaningful if the person does not want to color in the first place. Some activities may be structured (e.g., bingo) while others may be unstructured (e.g., staging an ice cream social, looking through magazines or cutting out coupons). Some may be passive (e.g., bird watching) and others may require a greater amount of physical effort (e.g., dancing or walking group). (Chapter 3 in this volume provides additional information on activities.) At the same time, the number of choices offered at one time should be somewhat limited, because too many choices can be overwhelming. The intent is to offer some choice to enhance residents' perceptions of control.

WHAT THE ENVIRONMENT CAN DO

Many options exist for increasing opportunities to exercise control in long-term care settings through physical features and spatial configurations. Some of the suggestions provided here have to do with enhancing control in the environment through private areas, orientation cues, greater choices, access to the outdoors, and room layouts. Other recommendations are related to providing spaces and features that support activity choices.

Private Areas

The environment can be made to appear more controllable by making it appear more manageable. This can be achieved by breaking up hallways so that they do not appear quite so long and endless. Nooks and alcoves along hallways and recessed doorways to bedrooms certainly can help. These also provide places for people to stop and rest if they wish to remove themselves from direct contact with other residents in hallways. If nooks, alcoves, and recesses do not exist in the facility and hallways are wider than the required minimum width imposed by state regulations, then seating and plants can be added to break up hallways.

Providing a space in the facility that can be used by residents when they are alone or with family also can help to control contact with others who may not be welcome during family visits. Most residents have come from their own homes, where they could determine with whom they spent time and how long visitors stayed. In shared residential settings, they literally are forced to spend time with any number of people they might not choose as friends, and often have few opportunities for retreat from these individuals. This type of private space may be especially important to residents who must share bedrooms (see Chapter 4 of this volume).

Choices

Design can contribute to perceptions of control when choices are available. For example, the ability to preview what is happening in a room before entering it allows residents the chance to decide whether they want to enter the room and participate in activities. This can be achieved when there are interior windows along a hallway wall. Those in the room also can observe what is happening elsewhere. Offering residents several colors to choose from when repainting bedrooms can provide residents with a greater sense of choice as well (see Chapter 2).

Some residents also may feel a greater sense of control when they can monitor the thermal comfort and lighting levels in their rooms. Easy-to-use, easy-to-read thermostats and light switches can facilitate this (see "Where to Find Products" later in this chapter). Even if residents can no longer set or adjust thermostats appropriately, having individual heating and air conditioning units for each room allows staff or families to set the temperatures to the resident's preferred setting. Many older people are sensitive to drafts and like the ambient temperature to be much warmer than what staff would prefer. In addition, certain physical features must be present before choices can even be offered. For example, tubs and showers must be present to offer residents the option of taking baths or showers.

Providing access to a variety of rooms probably offers the greatest amount of choice in the physical environment. Multiple rooms imply that different locations are available and opportunities exist to be alone or with others. Ideally, residents should also be able to choose between different-size groups. Multiple rooms that are distinct also enhance choice. Rooms can be distinct if they are of different sizes and have different decor, lighting, and furniture arrangements, and possibly even have different views to the outdoors. For example, one room might overlook a courtyard with a walking path while another might overlook large trees, providing residents with two different choices. Rooms also can differ depending on the type of activity that is taking place (busy/active or quiet/contemplative) and the decor. Having variety in furniture is important not only for the visual distinctiveness of rooms but also for accommodating a variety of residents. For example, not all people are the same size and shape, so one chair will not suit everyone. (Volume 2 covers this topic in more detail.) Ideally, residents should be able to bring in some of their own furniture to accommodate individual needs (Calkins, 1995).

Orientation Cues

If residents have difficulty finding their way around a building, then they may feel stressed and experience a diminished sense of control. One effective way to make a building easier to navigate is to create landmarks, or elements that create distinctive focal points. Some examples might be a large quilt hung on the wall, a large clock, birds in an aviary, or a fish aquarium (Figure 5.2). A large clock in a hallway, for example, might indicate that the dining room is a few feet ahead. Certain walls also might become landmarks if they are painted a distinctive color, although this may be less effective for residents with visual impairment or those who are color-blind. In addition, signage with large lettering on a contrasting background, photographs, or shadow boxes outside bedroom entries that document the history of the resident may help to create distinctive room entries. (Volume 2, Chapter 2 discusses orientation to place in more detail. Refer to "Where to Find Products" later in this section for sources for shadow boxes.)

Having purpose-specific rooms also can enhance orientation in buildings. Most older people lived in homes that had distinct living rooms, dining rooms, and kitchens that were used only for one purpose. In a similar manner, long-term care facilities should have rooms dedicated to specific purposes with visually distinct cues suggesting appropriate ways to act. A dining room that looks like a dining room and is used only for eating meals is an example. However, this is not always possible. A large dining room may be used for sing-alongs, socialization, and religious services between meals. Physical cues such as placing tablecloths on tables when it is time for a meal may help to minimize the confusion that can result from using rooms for multiple purposes.

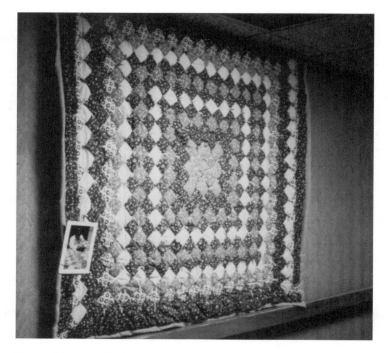

Figure 5.2.   A quilt hung on the wall in a hallway can provide a land-mark to help residents find their way around the facility.

Access to the Outdoors

In a study that addressed issues of autonomy for nursing facility residents who were cognitively intact (Kane & Freeman, n.d., cited in Walsh, 1990), the majority of residents indicated that freedom to leave the facility was their most important concern. Residents wanted to be able to leave for appointments or visits with family members. For residents with dementia, access to the outside is a bit more problematic. Although, for safety reasons, residents with dementia usually cannot be permitted to leave the facility whenever they wish, access to a secure outdoor space can support their sense of independence. Many residents may perceive themselves as still capable of living independently and do not realize that restrictions are in place for their own safety. An outdoor space that residents can freely access may help to provide residents with the perception that they have the opportunity to leave the unit even though they are still within the confines of the facility. This situation is much more desirable than simply restricting egress by securing or alarming all exit doors.

Activity Choices

The facility's environment must support activity choices. Within activity rooms, for example, there should be readily accessible storage for equipment and activity supplies. Spaces should be flexible to accommodate different types of activities or activities that are scheduled simultaneously. This can be accomplished by dividing the larger space into smaller, less overwhelming spaces with furniture and folding partition walls (see "Where to Find Products" for sources for dividers). A more permanent solution is the provision of half-walls, possibly with glass above them shielded by blinds or shades.

WHERE TO FIND PRODUCTS

Easy-to-See and Easy-to-Use Thermostats

Honeywell, Inc.
1985 Douglas Drive North
Golden Valley, MN 55422
(800) 345-6770, extension 7200
www.honeywell.com

Shadow Boxes

Exposures, Inc.
Post Office Box 3615
Oshkosh, WI 54903-3615
(800) 222-4947
www.exposuresonline.com
A catalog for the storage and display of photographs and mementos

Cabinets for Dividing Dining Rooms

Adden Furniture, Inc.
26 Jackson Street
Lowell, MA 01852
(508) 457-7848

Allsteel, Inc.
Allsteel Drive
Aurora, IL 60507
(800) 764-2535
www.allsteeloffice.com
Allsteel's InterChange panel system consists of dividers with acoustical inserts on both sides. The company also offers a variety of wheeled cabinets for storage.

♦ ♦ ♦

A summary sheet follows, which condenses the chapter text into a quick overview. The authors have also provided an area for you to make your own notes about your own staff and facility. Managerial staff may wish to use the summary sheets as handouts to accompany direct care staff training, or to post them by the time clock or nurses' station or include them in staff's pay envelopes.

AUTONOMY AND CONTROL SUMMARY SHEET

1. Control—when to get up, what to eat (imagine going to a restaurant and being told there was only one item on the menu for dinner), how to arrange your furniture, who to spend time with, when to be alone—is something most people highly prize and value.
2. Physical and sensory changes may reduce autonomy. For instance, impaired hearing makes it hard to hear and make sense of conversations. It can also limit the number of places you can go where you can hear and understand what is going on.
3. Residents' autonomy is often sacrificed for concern over safety and well-being. For instance, residents may not be allowed outside for fear that they may fall or may not be allowed to skip breakfast, even though they have never been breakfast eaters.

What Staff Can Do

1. Allow residents to alter or arrange their spaces to the greatest extent possible.
2. Respect residents' wishes when they say no.
3. Ask residents' preference before providing assistance. Ask whether they want milk in their coffee today, even when you know this is their preference.
4. Give residents two or three pieces of clothing to choose between instead of making the choice for them.
5. Work to develop policies that allow residents to wake up and go to bed when they want to.

What the Environment Can Do

1. When all of the residents' rooms are alike, there is little choice or meaning in being in one space over another. Therefore, different rooms and spaces should be *different*— in size, decor, and function.
2. A well-designed, safe outdoor space that is directly adjacent to the unit, which staff can easily see into should be created. Allow residents unrestricted access to this space.
3. Seating in both sun and shade should be provided.
4. Having a kitchen on the unit makes it easier to let residents rise when they want because it allows staff to offer a continental breakfast to both the early and the late risers. It also makes it easier to offer an alternative meal if a resident does not like the meal being served.

YOUR NOTES

6
Residential Design

Naomi has just started looking for a residential long-term care facility for her mother. It is important to Naomi that the facility be as much like home as possible. Although her mother has dementia and needs some help that Naomi cannot provide, she is not happy about having to move from a house she has been living in for 45 years. Naomi believes that a homelike facility will help to minimize the trauma and disruption of her mother's future move.

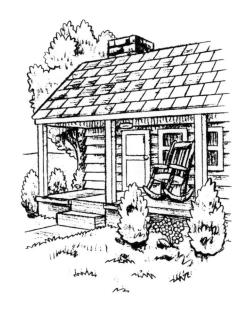

Naomi walks into one prospective facility and is astounded by the beauty of the front room. Everything is well coordinated, and the furniture looks expensive and elegant, yet she cannot imagine her mother in such a place. She has had the same living room furniture for 20 years and likes to take naps on the couch. Naomi is sure that no one ever takes naps on the sofas in this front room. She enters a second facility and cannot believe how large the space is. It is two or three stories high, and there are lots of skylights and hanging plants. Signage with many arrows points to different locations. Naomi feels a little confused: Is this an atrium in a mall or the lobby of a grand hotel? Naomi can just imagine how much more confused her mother would be if she were to move into such a place. Naomi *walks into a third facility and is surprised that the corridor from the lobby has bedrooms on both sides. Where is the living room or dining room? Eventually, she reaches a day room at the end of the corridor that has similar institutional-looking chairs lined up against the back wall. Naomi cannot bear the thought of her mother sitting in one of those chairs and quickly leaves.*

Finding a residential or homelike long-term care facility can be a difficult task because creating homelike settings is not as easy as one might think (Calkins, 1995). This chapter offers design suggestions for enhancing residential character in existing long-term care settings. Specifically, the recommendations address physical modifications to the environment, including the spatial adjacencies of the different rooms in a facility, the scale of rooms, the use of rooms, and the decor of the spaces, including finishes, furnishings, and lighting.

WHAT THE ENVIRONMENT CAN DO

Spatial Adjacencies

When you go home this evening and open the front door to your home, you will not walk right into your bedroom. You will probably enter a foyer, some sort of vestibule, or your living room. Most American homes are designed so that the front door faces the street and leads to the more public areas of a house. Semipublic spaces, such as the living room and dining room, are typically located toward the front of the house, are a bit more formal, and are used for entertaining friends and acquaintances. If you were to open the back door to your home this evening instead, you would probably enter your kitchen or perhaps a family room. Again, you would not walk right into your bedroom. The back door of an American house typically is accessed from a back or side yard or a garage and leads to the less formal spaces of a house. The kitchen, for example, is used for meal preparation and informal family gatherings. To get to the more private rooms of your house, you probably would have to enter some sort of transitional space such as a hallway off the kitchen or family room. This transitional space helps to separate the bedrooms from the other rooms in the house. If the bedrooms are located on the second floor, then you will have to climb a staircase, another transitional element.

In contrast, the vast majority of long-term care facilities are arranged so that the entrance to the unit leads directly to a hallway of bedrooms. The long hallway with bedrooms on both sides has been used over and over again as the most economical way to organize space for large numbers of people. A day room or lounge, used for dining as well as activities, often is provided at the end of the hallway so that residents and visitors must pass by private bedrooms to get to the more public common area. These hallways can be as long as 50 feet. This type of arrangement can be difficult to navigate and can be unfamiliar to residents with dementia after identifying with the typical layout of a house for most of their lives. Facilities should not be restricted by this arrangement. Existing long-term care facilities and those considering new construction can incorporate the spatial adjacencies that would typically be encountered in a house in several ways.

Reorganize Spaces

Most facilities are restricted by their existing floor plan and cannot afford to remodel extensively, but spaces can be added or reorganized to incorporate some of the spatial adjacencies of a house (Figure 6.1). For example, many facilities have recognized the benefits of having a kitchen or partial kitchen on each unit. A kitchen can be added adjacent to the dining area (often a day room). A small foyer at the entrance to the unit with a small closet for coats and hats can be created to provide residents and visitors with a transitional entry space (Calkins, 1995). If it is feasible to rearrange or add plumbing, then it may be possible to relocate the more public areas of the unit closer to the entrance by converting the day room/lounge, typically at the end of a long hallway, into one or two resident rooms. Two existing resident bedrooms at the entrance to the unit then can be turned into living and dining rooms.

Plan for Adjacencies

For facilities considering new construction in the future, there are greater opportunities for incorporating the spatial adjacencies of the house into a long-term care design. In one facility in particular, The Wealshire, located outside of Chicago, great effort was made to create the spatial feeling of a house (Figure 6.2). The Wealshire is a 144-bed rest home and skilled nursing facility comprising many households of 18 residents each. Each household consists of a front entrance, off an enclosed front yard, that immediately opens into a living room as in a typical house. An adjacent dining room is separated from the living room by a bakers' rack, which allows staff to monitor both rooms visually from various points. As with a typical house, there is also a back door that opens into a back hall with a coat closet. This transitional hall leads into the kitchen. Short hallways lead to the more private rooms, which are bedrooms,

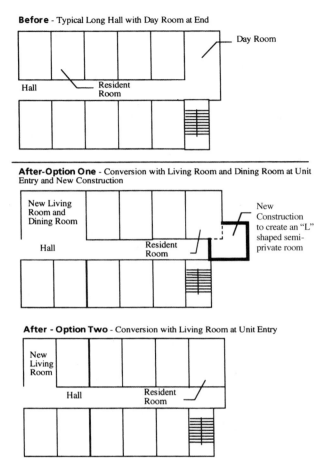

Figure 6.1.   Ways to reorganize spaces within a facility to incorporate the spatial adjacencies of a typical American house.

and a staff work area is located at the intersection of the two hallways for visual monitoring. Such spatial adjacencies can be incorporated during the project conceptualization or schematic design phase.

Scale

Homes have a certain scale. Most rooms are one story, with ceiling heights extending anywhere from 8 to 10 feet. The living room or family room is typi-

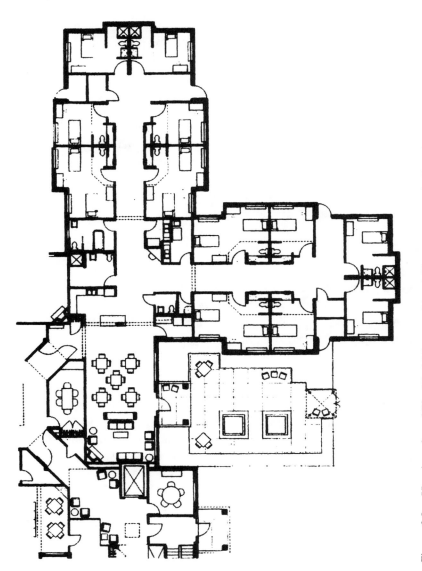

Figure 6.2. Housing plan of The Wealshire, a residential long-term care facility whose units have been constructed to resemble the spatial layout of a typical American house.

cally the largest room in a house, but it rarely exceeds 300 square feet. The hallway to the bedrooms is probably less than 15 feet in length and is 3–4 feet wide. More than likely, the windows are somewhere between 2 and 4 feet wide; there are no huge panes of glass from floor to ceiling.

In contrast, many long-term care facilities have large living rooms that are two stories in height and resemble the size and scale of a hotel lobby. Similarly, dining rooms are often more like what would be encountered in a large restaurant, and hallways can appear long and endless as in many hotels. This disparity in scale is partly because most homes are designed to house one family consisting of a few people, whereas most long-term care facilities must accommodate 20, 60, or even 100 people. The large scale of existing long-term care facilities can be difficult to resolve. Nevertheless, there are ways to break up the apparent scale of hallways and large spaces. For those facilities considering new construction, clustering spaces can be a way to reduce scale and to create a more familiar, homelike size. This is discussed in more detail in the following text.

Break Up Scale of Long Hallways

Long hallways not only appear institutional but they can require a great deal of energy for older people to walk through and can be difficult to navigate if the doorways on both sides look similar. Several techniques can be used to break up long hallways. First, doorways can be distinguished from one another. For example, more important doorways, such as the entrance to a bathroom, can be decorated with a three-dimensional canopy that can be seen from down the hall (Figure 6.3). Residents' bedroom doors can be painted a resident's favorite color or decorated with favorite pieces of art. Personal cues such as a display case with photographs can be placed outside entry doors. These strategies not only help to break up hallways but they also help to provide orientation cues. Second, unique landmarks such as a grandfather clock, a chest of drawers, a large colorful quilt, or textured artwork can provide visual and tactile interest as well as orienting cues. Third, if hallways are wider than the required minimum width imposed by state regulations (often 8 feet), small seating areas can be placed along the path to give residents the opportunity to rest or socialize. (Volume 2 covers many of these issues in more depth.)

Break Up Scale of Large Spaces

Large spaces can appear institutional and can be overwhelming and intimidating for residents with dementia. Smaller spaces are more residential and can be conducive to conversation. This is particularly important for dining

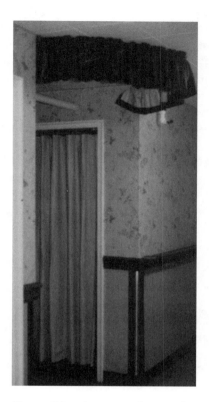

Figure 6.3. A canopy that can be seen from down the hall is useful for residents to distinguish important doorways, such as the entrance to a bathroom.

rooms and activity rooms. It is best to have several small dining rooms for 5–10 people or several small activity rooms, such as a library or crafts rooms, but few facilities can afford this luxury. However, this effect can be achieved in multiple ways. If a space is used only for dining, for example, then permanent dividers can be constructed. These dividers can be attractive short walls with planters or latticework hanging above them. It is often beneficial to look at the ways in which restaurants create smaller areas without completely dividing a space. Dividers, possibly with built-in shelves for storage, can be used to create smaller spaces to accommodate different types of activities.

If a large space is used for multiple activities, then it may be possible to divide the space into smaller areas perceptually or functionally with moveable screens. These screens can consist of standard panelized screens found at most home decorating stores. The facility also can make screens by using two-way hinges and shutters or pieces of plywood. Screens should be at least 5 feet tall to block the vision of those who are seated and to diffuse some sound. Where storage is a concern, especially in activity areas, a large space can be divided into smaller areas temporarily with large storage cabinets with locking casters (see "Where to Find Products" later in this chapter for sources). The facility also can purchase wardrobe cabinets and attach casters to them. When the large space is needed for special holiday meals or activities, such as concerts for large groups, the cabinets or screens can be moved against the wall. In addition, furniture can be arranged in small groupings. Such an arrangement helps divide a room into smaller areas and encourages socialization at the same time.

Cluster Spaces

For new construction, clustering spaces into smaller "households" of 10–20 residents can reduce the scale of one large building and provide a more familiar size. Within each household, clustering bedrooms around central living spaces such as a dining room and living room is a more residential pattern than the traditional nursing facility design, in which long hallways radiate off a nurses' station (see Figure 6.1). The smaller scale of clusters helps to define a comfortable group size for social interaction and organized activities. In addition, the scale of individual rooms can appear more manageable if ceiling heights are low—8 or 9 feet high.

Purpose-Specific Rooms

Most of us have a separate living room, dining room, kitchen, and family room in our own homes. Each room has a distinct character and is used for a specific purpose. The dining room, for example, may be used for large family dinners or for dinner parties with friends. The kitchen may be large enough for the immediate family to eat informally or to casually gather during meal preparation. That does not mean that we do not spread our bills out over the dining room table or our children do not do their homework there. We also engage in many types of activities in a multipurpose family room. In general, however, various cues indicate what types of behaviors are appropriate in each space, and specific activities occur in each room. This was especially true for the previous homes of many older adults who are in their 80s and 90s and living in long-term care settings.

In contrast, many long-term care facilities have multipurpose rooms that are used for dining and for various large group activities such as holiday celebrations or church services. They also have day rooms, lounges, craft rooms, and tub rooms. These types of spaces can be utterly confusing for residents with dementia, who may not be able to determine what behaviors are appropriate in such unfamiliar spaces as day rooms. Fortunately, there are many ways, using both terminology and cues, in which existing long-term care facilities can provide purpose-specific rooms.

Use Residential Language

Rooms can be identified using terminology that older adults would have encountered in their previous homes. For example, staff can refer to day rooms and lounges as living rooms or dining rooms. Corridors can be called halls or hallways, and different activity rooms can be designated as libraries, television rooms, or music rooms. In addition, nurses' work areas can be incorporated within kitchen areas or included within separate rooms labeled as offices.

Use Familiar Cues

Residents will be able to recognize a dining room as a dining room more easily if this space looks like a dining room and is used only for meal-related purposes such as setting the table, eating, chatting over coffee, or cleaning up. Smaller family-size dining rooms with four- to six-person tables that are used only for meal-related purposes are ideal. However, many facilities are restricted by their existing floor plan and must work with large spaces that support many different kinds of activities. In such cases, a series of familiar cues can be developed that identify when a space is being used as a dining room. For instance, setting tables or having some residents help set the tables with placemats and silverware will let residents know that it is almost time for a meal. Olfactory cues can help as well. Most of us are used to smelling a meal as it is cooked at home. Although most facilities will not be able to cook all or part of a meal on the unit, brewing coffee and baking rolls or cookies in a toaster oven just before serving meals can provide cues for residents. Also try to serve at least one meal family-style if state codes permit. If this is not possible, then serving food on plates instead of institutional trays is much more reminiscent of eating at home.

Familiar cues are important in other rooms as well. If a unit is fortunate enough to have several shared social spaces, then the facility's goal should be to make each one distinct, and similar to a room that would be found in a resident's house. The label or term *family room,* for example, connotes a certain image. A family room in a long-term care facility should be comfortable, with couches and pillows, and filled with the sounds of a television or a radio. A living room should be a bit more formal, with more elegant furniture and knickknacks. In contrast, the term *day room* conjures images of chairs lined up around the perimeter of the room and a cacophony of call bells, alarms, and a public address system. This could be confusing for residents with dementia.

Decor

Think about your own home again. You probably have a couch that is upholstered with a patterned fabric in your living room rather than several metal chairs with vinyl cushions. You may have a bed with a wooden headboard or brass posts rather than a hospital bed. You may also have lamps on nightstands rather than fluorescent lighting hanging over your bed. In addition, you probably decorated your home over several years, collecting furnishings a few pieces at a time as you could afford them, selecting new carpeting for each room as old ones became worn or too dirty to shampoo, and painting or wallpapering as your tastes and fashions changed. The finishes and furnishings you selected, as well as the eclectic process of decorating that is typical for most people, often lead to a certain homelike look and a comfortable feeling. In other words, your home probably is not overly decorated or picture perfect; and you usually feel as if you can put your feet on the coffee table or take a nap on the couch in the living room.

In contrast, some long-term care facilities have furnishings and finishes that contribute to an institutional decor. Metal blinds on windows, metal frame chairs, shiny vinyl flooring, and blank walls usually evoke images of institutions. Other facilities hire interior decorators or designers, who often want to overdecorate and overcoordinate. The result can be beautiful; many of these facilities look as if they could be featured in the shelter magazines *Architectural Digest* or *Metropolitan Home.* Yet the majority of older adults did not live in such houses before relocating to a nursing facility. Many long-term care settings also look like grand hotels or corporate offices. They have a commercial look that is not typical of most homes in the United States.

When providing decor in long-term care facilities that is more like home, certain types of finishes, furnishings, window treatments, accessories, and lighting should be taken into account. These features not only should be residential in character but they also should enhance function and include materials that are durable enough to withstand routine cleaning and use by

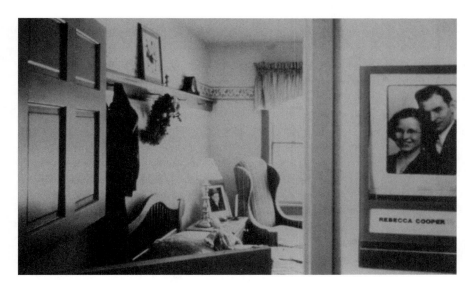

Figure 6.4.   Incorporating a resident's personal possessions and allowing the resident to select the decor can make the bedroom more like home.

many people. These features are discussed here in relation to the different spaces in a facility, including resident bedrooms and bathrooms, dining rooms, tub rooms, hallways, and kitchens. A number of recommendations are drawn from the book *Designing for Alzheimer's Disease: Strategies for Creating Better Care Environments* (Brawley, 1997).

Residents' Bedrooms

Residents' bedrooms are often the most personal areas in long-term care facilities. Ideally, residents should be able to bring personal possessions from their previous homes and arrange furniture, hang artwork, and select decor, including paint colors, window treatments, and bedspreads, as they like (Figure 6.4). Fire regulation codes, however, may restrict residents from bringing in certain pieces of upholstered furniture as well as bedspreads and drapery fabrics (see Chapter 2 of this volume). When this is not possible, residential-style furnishings and finishes should be incorporated.

If hospital beds are required in state codes, then some companies can modify hospital beds with headboards and footboards. It is important to provide appropriate and supportive beds that look residential (see "Where to Find Products" at the end of this chapter for sources). It is also important to specify twin beds if single beds are provided in a long-term care facility be-cause dormitory beds often are selected instead. Dormitory beds are longer than twin beds and are not as wide. This unfamiliar size can be disconcerting to residents with dementia, who may be adjusting to sleeping in smaller beds (Brawley, 1997).

Nightstands and dressers should be made of wood. Drawer pulls and handles should be easy to manipulate even for people with limited agility in their hands. Generally, C-shaped handles are easier to grasp than small knobs. Glide surfaces should be free of dirt and oiled regularly to maximize opera-tion. If a chair is provided in the bedroom, then it should be made of wood and fabric (as opposed to a metal frame and vinyl). (Refer to "Where to Find Products" for information on residential-style furniture.) Televisions should be placed in a location where glare from windows is not reflected onto television screens. If possible, furniture arrangements in bedrooms should be similar to the way in which furniture was arranged in residents' previous homes. This helps residents to get around their rooms without bumping into furniture.

In addition, a grooming area in the bedroom may help to enhance a homelike feeling because a dressing table is found in many homes. Many res-idents may not be able to stand in front of a mirror for a long period of time or may not be accustomed to grooming themselves while seated on their beds. The grooming area can be as simple as providing a small table and mirror with adequate lighting as well as a chair. Brushes, combs, and other items can be placed on the table within easy reach. If this is not possible because of space limitations, then consider creating such a place in the tub room (Figure 6.5).

Residential finishes, including wall and ceiling finishes and floor cov-erings, are also important. If walls are painted rather than wallpapered, then flat paint should be used because this decreases the amount of reflected glare. When selecting paint colors, you might want to consider colors that were pop-ular among residents in their previous homes. A survey of older adults in cen-tral Ohio long-term care facilities (Zavotka & Teaford, 1998) revealed that brown, yellow, blue, and green are the colors that were used most often in the homes in which older adults lived before moving into a long-term care facil-ity. Using these colors, at least in Ohio facilities, could be a familiar cue for older people and would not be much more expensive than the various shades of white and beige or the latest trendy, fashionable colors that typically are used. Color contrast should also be considered to distinguish walls from floors and to distinguish between furniture and the background (walls and floors). For example, consider a darker wall and a light-colored floor.

Wall paint colors can be used in conjunction with a variety of wallpa-per and border patterns. These do not have to be extremely well coordinated

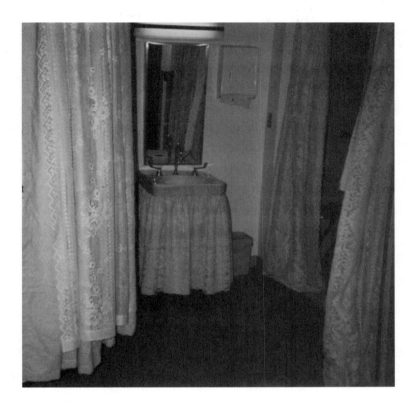

Figure 6.5. A grooming area like this one can be created in the tub room.

because most people did not live in homes that could appear in a magazine layout. Although no research dealing with patterns exists, and we do not know which patterns work best with residents with dementia, there is some anecdotal evidence that residents may become dizzy or disoriented by large geometric patterns, may experience unsteadiness with wavy or undulating patterns, or may misperceive stripes as bars. These problems are likely to be pronounced when the contrast in the patterning is high. In general, small, classic patterns are preferable to contemporary ones.

With respect to floor coverings, carpeting is ideal as a residential finish. Carpeting has several advantages over resilient flooring (Wise, 1996). First, it is more residential in appearance. It is less slippery when liquids are spilled, and therefore less likely to cause a fall. When falls do occur, there are fewer injuries associated with falls on carpeting, particularly if it has a cushioned backing, than on resilient flooring. Carpeting significantly reduces glare. Using carpeting can also reduce background noise. Studies have shown that background noise can be diminished by 70% when carpeting is added (Baucom, 1996). Finally, there is some evidence that, although carpeting may have a higher initial cost than resilient flooring, it is less expensive to maintain and therefore has a lower life-cycle cost (see "Where to Find Products" for carpeting sources). When selecting carpeting, be sure to look for the following features:

- Loop construction
- High density (4,000 fibers per square yard) with low pile height (¼–⅜ inch)
- Heavy weight (22–26 ounces face weight)
- Solution-dyed fibers
- Solid/moisture-proof backing and welded seams
- Inherent antimicrobial treatment (lasts longer than surface-applied treatments)
- No borders or patterns with high contrast
- Emissions and off-gassing that is low enough to meet the Carpet and Rug Institute's Indoor Air Quality test

Accessories such as bedspreads, window curtains, artwork, throw pillows, and natural plants can contribute to a homelike feeling as well. Many institutional environments are filled with hard, sterile surfaces; accessories can add softness and texture. As with wallpaper and border patterns, small, classic patterns are recommended for bedspreads, window curtains, and throw pillows. Pillows of different shapes, sizes, and textures should have covers that can be easily removed and laundered. Window sheers are not only more residential looking than blinds, they also allow light to be diffused without totally blocking views. In contrast, vertical and horizontal blinds create slits of light and dark, which can be disorienting to residents with dementia. The bright colors, textures, and fragrances of plants can brighten a room. Although natural plants are much more desirable than silk plants, residents with middle-stage and late-stage dementia often put things in their mouths, including plants. Staff should make sure that all plants are nontoxic (Brawley, 1997; see the list of toxic plants in Appendix C).

Finding a balance between non–institutional-looking and functional lighting can be challenging. Wall-mounted fluorescent lights that are placed over a bed should not be used in residents' bedrooms. They are clinical in appearance, and fluorescent lights often have extremely bright and unshielded bulbs that produce glare, shadows, and uneven lighting. There should be enough and different types of lighting (e.g., overhead and task lighting). Task lighting is usually provided by table or floor lamps in most homes and should be used in resident bedrooms. (Volume 2 covers lighting from a functional standpoint in much more detail. See "Where to Find Products" at the end of the chapter for sources of various types of lighting.)

Residents' Bathrooms

As with resident bedrooms, finishes in individual bathrooms should be residential in nature. To help residents maintain continence, however, color contrast is important in this room. Bathroom walls and floors should be a different color from the fixtures so that the fixtures stand out. If this is not possible, then the color of the toilet seat should be dark so that the toilet, if it is a light color, is more prominent. Adding borders, decorative towels, plants that do well in moist environments, and curtains around windows or under sinks can also help to enhance the residential character.

Tub Room

There are times when residents must use the tub room. Resident bathrooms may not include a tub or shower area, and some residents may need assistance with bathing. Often, the tub room is one of the most institutional looking rooms in the facility. Yet bathing can be a more pleasurable experience when environmental modifications are made to the tub room to enhance residential character (Figure 6.6). Wallpaper and border patterns, colorful towels, and patterned curtains around windows, tubs, or even under sinks can be used. Decor that is moisture resistant or plasticized will hold up longer. Plants that do well in a moist atmosphere can be added as well (a grow light will be needed if the tub room has no windows). These sound-absorbing items will help to decrease the excess background noise that occurs in rooms with hard surfaces. Softer lighting, such as cove lighting, also can add to a residential character. In addition, a grooming area with a vanity, seat, and mirror can be incorporated within the tub room if space is not available in resident bedrooms or private bathrooms. This can be achieved simply by providing a table with a skirt and a mirror.

Dining Rooms

The dining room was a part of the home where women residents in particular spent many hours. Their dining rooms probably were filled with family

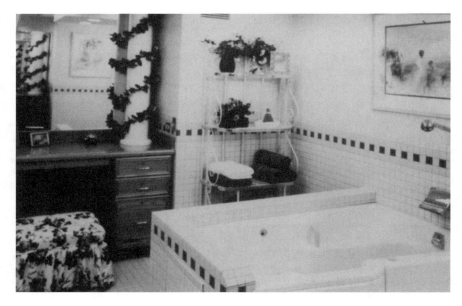

Figure 6.6.   Modification of a tub room using a vanity, shelving, and plants can minimize its institutional look.

heirlooms and treasures. A hutch or china cabinet may have been used to display china, silver, or glassware handed down for generations. Ideally, residents should be encouraged to personalize shared spaces in the facility with these personal possessions from previous homes to reflect their identities (see Chapter 2 for additional information). Reflecting identities, however, can be difficult in a group living arrangement. Issues of territoriality may arise with regard to furniture, and residents and family members may not feel comfortable placing furnishings or objects of even modest economic or sentimental value in a public place. In this case, the facility may have to purchase furnishings and decorate shared spaces.

If the facility is considering buying new furniture, a number of manufacturers make commercial-grade, highly durable dining room furniture that looks residential (see "Where to Find Products" for sources). It is beneficial to purchase furniture that is somewhat similar to the furniture that residents would bring into a facility in terms of the types of pieces purchased and the style of the furniture. For example, items such as china cabinets or hutches with dishes displayed add a residential feeling. Furnishings do not have to

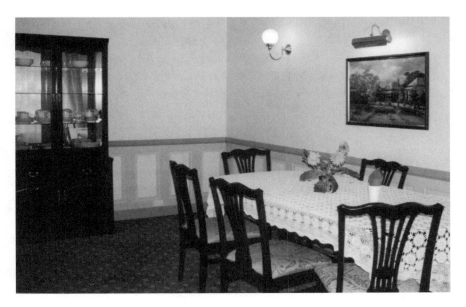

Figure 6.7.   Dining rooms look more homelike with the addition of residential-style furniture, carpeting, lighting, and wall finishes.

match exactly in terms of wood type, wood or fabric color, and pattern. In other words, the dining room should not be overdecorated. An eclectic look with many different but coordinated pieces of furniture is much more like the homes with which older adults have identified over a lifetime (Figure 6.7).

When buying new furniture for a dining room, the facility must consider a number of functional issues. (These issues are addressed only briefly here because functional requirements and dimensions for furniture are covered in detail in Volume 2, Chapter 5.) Square tables usually are best because each resident is provided with a clearly defined eating territory. Bullnose or round-edged treatments are more comfortable to rest against than are sharp edges. Tables with contrasting edges, through the use of a different color or material, are easier for residents to see. Tabletops made of wood or wood laminates are warm and familiar to residents and should have a matte finish to reduce glare. Avoid the use of polishes or coatings that are highly reflective. The use of tablecloths during meals provides a residential feeling, but the color should contrast with dishes or individual place mats and the floor covering. Tables with four legs tend to be more sturdy and familiar to residents than tables with a center pedestal. However, pedestal tables are easier to use with wheelchairs, and often the bases of pedestal tables can be adjusted in height to accommodate both wheelchair and conventional chair users.

When selecting residential-style chairs, make sure that chair arms fit under the table so that residents can get close enough to the table. Chair arms are essential and should extend beyond the front edge of the seat. This enables residents to use the arms for support when rising. Casters on two of the chair legs make it easier for residents to pull up to and push back from tables. Glides, which are metal disks attached to chair legs, also make it easier to move chairs.

With respect to finishes, carpeting in a dining room is residential looking, and it can withstand staining and maintain its appearance. It requires routine and scheduled maintenance, but so do resilient floors, which often are mopped after every meal. As with resident bedrooms, paint colors can be used in conjunction will wallpaper and border patterns. Details such as low-cost wood moldings (e.g., crown molding, chair rails, and bases) as well as wainscoting, provide a familiar residential character (check with your local home improvement warehouse or lumber mill for sources). Plants and flower arrangements in the centers of tables also can brighten dining rooms.

Dining rooms in long-term care facilities tend to be large, open rooms, making them difficult to light well. To achieve adequate lighting, an ambient lighting system should be used in combination with decorative lighting (Brawley, 1997). Ambient light can be provided by cove lighting, a method of indirect lighting in which the light source is attached to the wall and is directed up to a reflective surface. Chandeliers or other pendant lighting hung from the ceiling surface tend to be decorative and residential looking and provide direct lighting. "These should be located above eye level and frosted, filament-wrapped, or shaded bulbs should be used to control glare" (Brawley, 1997, p. 166). This type of direct lighting works best with ceiling heights above 8 feet. Adjustable lighting controls are advantageous; lighting can be turned up during breakfast hours and then turned down at lunchtime if there is a great deal of natural light. (Volume 2, Chapter 5 covers lighting in dining rooms in much more detail. Sources for various types of lighting are provided in "Where to Find Products" at the end of this chapter.)

Therapeutic Kitchens

The kitchen is often the center of the home. For many older women, the kitchen is a familiar and comfortable environment. Providing at least a small therapeutic kitchen on a unit for residents to use may help enhance residential

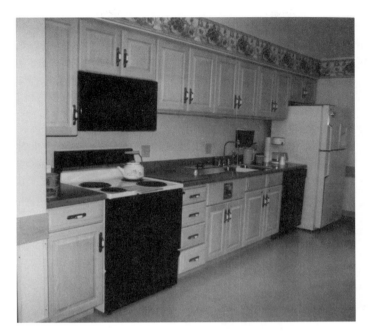

Figure 6.8. A therapeutic kitchen can be furnished with most of the appliances, storage cabinets, and work surfaces that are found in a typical American home.

character. Sinks, refrigerators, stoves, cabinets, and countertops that typically would be found in most homes should be used (Figure 6.8). Because stoves raise safety concerns, they should have a hidden power switch that automatically turns off the appliance after a certain amount of time.

Kitchen cabinets should be wood or wood laminate, a familiar residential material. Wall-mounted cabinets should be lowered several inches so that short residents, residents in wheelchairs, and residents with a limited range of motion can reach them more easily. Accessories can include canister sets, potholders, cookie jars, bread boxes, or other familiar kitchen items. Flooring rather than carpeting typically is associated with kitchens in most homes. Resilient flooring can be used, including sheet vinyl or vinyl composition tile. However, flooring should not be shiny, even though many long-term care facilities associate shiny floors with their being clean. Shiny floors can be a source of indirect glare. (See "Where To Find Products" for sources of nonglare resilient flooring.)

WHERE TO FIND PRODUCTS

Cabinets for Dividing Rooms

Adden Furniture, Inc.
26 Jackson Street
Lowell, MA 01852
(508) 457-7848

Allsteel, Inc.
Allsteel Drive
Aurora, IL 60507
(800) 764-2535
www.allsteeloffice.com
Allsteel's InterChange panel system consists of dividers with acoustical inserts on both sides. The company also offers a variety of wheeled cabinets for storage.

Residential-Style Furniture

Adjustable-Height Tables

Falcon Products, Inc.
9387 Dielman Industrial Drive
St. Louis, MO 63132-2214
(800) 8873-3252
www.falconproducts.com
Access adjustable-height dining room table bases

Johnson Tables
1424 Davis Road
Elgin, IL 60123
(800) 346-5555

Kimball Lodging Group
1180 East 16th Street
Jasper, IN 47549-1009
(800) 451-8090
www.lodging.kimball.com
Health care and hospitality furniture

Space Tables
8035 Ranchers Road NE
Post Office Box 32082
Minneapolis, MN 55432-0082
(800) 328-2580
www.spacetables.com

Dining Room Chairs

HumanCare
14930 South Main Street
Gardena, CA 90248
(800) 767-4001
Human Care manufactures a variety of seating styles; custom seat heights can be special ordered.

Lifespan
5901 Christie Avenue, Suite 101
Emeryville, CA 94608
(510) 601-6275
www.furnishings.com

Sauder Manufacturing
930 West Barre Road
Archbold, OH 43502-0230
(800) 537-1530
www.saudermanufacturing.com
Sauder offers a variety of health care-seating products.

Additional Furniture

American of Martinsville
128 East Church Street
Martinsville, VA 24112
(540) 632-2061
www.americanofmartinsville.com

Basic American Medical Products
2935-A Northeast Parkway
Atlanta, GA 30360-2048
(770) 368-4700
www.basicamerican.com

Carroll Healthcare
1881 Huron Street
London, Ontario N5V 3A5, Canada
(800) 668-2337
www.carrollhealthcare.com

Duraframe
Post Office Box 1870
Ridgeland, SC 29936
(800) 405-3441
www.duraframe.com

Healthcare Furnishings, Inc.
31 Innwood Circle, Suite 109
Little Rock, AR 72211
(800) 648-5744
www.healthcarefurnishings.com

Invacare Continuing Care Group
739 Goddard Avenue
Chesterfield, MO 63005
(800) 347-5440
www.invacare-ccg.com

Kimball Healthcare
1600 Royal Street
Jasper, IN 47549-1001
(800) 482-1616
www.kimball.com

NOA Medical Industries
801 Terry Lane
Washington, MO 63090
(800) 633-6068
www.noamedical.com

Primarily Seating
475 Park Avenue, Suite 3A
New York, NY 10022
(212) 838-2588
www.primarilyseating.com

Town Square
Post Office Box 419
Hillsboro, TX 76645
(800) 345-1663
www.gliderrocker.com

Carpeting

Bonar Floors
365 Walt Sanders Memorial Drive
Newnan, GA 30265
(770) 252-4890
www.bonarfloors.com

Collins & Aikman Floorcoverings, Inc.
311 Smith Industrial Boulevard
Dalton, GA 30722-1447
(800) 248-2878
www.powerbond.com

Interface Flooring System, Inc.
Post Office Box 1503
LaGrange, GA 30241
Tiles for health care facilities; carpeting that is antimicrobial and, because of Interface's solid backing system, can be easily repaired by cutting out stains.

Lees Commercial Carpets
3330 West Friendly Avenue
Post Office Box 26027
Greensboro, NC 27410
(800) 523-5647

Lowes Carpet Corporation
160 Duvall Road
Chatsworth, GA 30705
(800) 333-2468

Lighting

Lighting Consultants

Eunice Noell-Waggoner
Center for Design for an Aging Society
6200 S.W. Virginia Avenue, Suite 210
Portland, OR 97201
(503) 246-8231
Noell-Waggoner is an expert in the field of lighting for aging people.

Illuminating Engineering Society of North America
120 Wall Street, Floor 17
New York, NY 10005
(212) 248-5000
www.iesna.org
Lighting and the Visual Environment for Senior Living (1998)

Lighthouse International
111 East 59th Street
New York, NY 10022-1202
(800) 829-0500
www.lighthouse.org
Offers a variety of solutions and products for individuals with visual impairment

Lighting Resources

Architectural Lighting Systems
30 Sherwood Drive
Taunton, MA 02780
(508) 823-8277
Cove lighting manufacturer

Holophane Co.
214 Oakwood Avenue
Newark, OH 43055
Baffles for fluorescent lights

Microsun, Inc.
(800) 657-0077
www.microsun.com
Floor and table lamps that use combination incandescent and metal halide lamps to provide high-efficiency, high-level lighting

Schumaker Lighting, Inc.
Adjustable Fixture Co.
3726 North Booth Street
Milwaukee, WI 53223-4714
(800) 558-2628
www.adjustablefixture.com

SPI Lighting Inc.
10400 North Enterprise Drive
Mequon, WI 53092
(414) 242-1420
www.spilighting.com

Dining Room Furniture

Adjustable-Height Tables

Falcon Products, Inc.
9387 Dielman Industrial Drive
St. Louis, MO 63132-2214
(800) 873-3252
www.falconproducts.com
Adjustable-height dining room table bases

Johnson Tables
1424 Davis Road
Elgin, IL 60123
(800) 346-5555

Kimball Lodging Group
1180 East 16th Street
Jasper, IN 47549-1009
(800) 451-8090
www.lodging.kimball.com
Health care and hospitality furniture

Space Tables
8035 Ranchers Road NE
Post Office Box 32082
Minneapolis, MN 55432-0082
(800) 328-2580
www.spacetables.com

Dining Room Chairs

HumanCare
14930 South Main Street
Gardena, CA 90248
(800) 767-4001
Offers a variety of seating styles; custom seat heights can be special ordered

Lifespan
5901 Christie Avenue, Suite 101
Emeryville, CA 94608
(510) 601-6275
www.furnishings.com

Sauder Manufacturing
930 West Barre Road
Archbold, OH 43502-0230
(800) 537-1530
www.saudermanufacturing.com
A variety of health care-seating products

Nonglare Resilient Flooring

Mannington Mills, Inc.
Post Office Box 30
Salem, NJ 08079
(800) 356-6787
www.mannington.com

TOLI International
55 Mall Drive
Commack, NY 11725
(800) 446-5476
www.toli.com
Vinyl sheets and vinyl tile that are extremely durable and have a variety
of hardwood floor appearances; These products also have less sheen as
compared with other vinyl flooring

♦ ♦ ♦

A summary sheet follows, which condenses the chapter text into a
quick overview. The authors have also provided an area for you to make your
own notes about your own staff and facility. Managerial staff may wish to use
the summary sheets as handouts to accompany direct care staff training, or to
post them by the time clock or nurses' station or include them in staff's pay
envelopes.

RESIDENTIAL DESIGN SUMMARY SHEET

1. Being surrounded by personal belongings helps residents to feel comfortable and at home.

What Staff Can Do

1. Arrange furniture in small groupings, with chairs at right angles, to support conversation. This configuration is more familiar to residents than having furniture arranged around the perimeter of the room.
2. Add pretty, decorative touches to bath and tub rooms.
3. Laminate photographs or prints so that they do not get wet in the steam that comes from the bath or shower.
4. Add an attractively decorated shelf.
5. Add wallpaper border or trim, or stick-on decorations for bath tiles.
6. Add plants that like moist areas, such as ferns. These plants often do well in bathrooms when there is natural light.

What the Environment Can Do

1. Create spaces that look and feel familiar to residents. Rooms that look like what residents had at home can cue residents to appropriate behavior. Language, or what you call the room, is also important. Avoid the use of terms such as *day room*.
2. Break up the scale of larger rooms by using furniture as dividers. If there is money in the budget, then purchase wardrobes on locking castor wheels. These can be used to subdivide a space.
3. Encourage residents to bring personal possessions, including furniture, art, and knickknacks, from home to be placed in the shared areas of the unit.

YOUR NOTES

Bibliography

Alzheimer's Association. (1997). *Key elements of dementia care.* Chicago: Author.

Baucom, A.H. (1996). *Hospitality design: For the graying generation.* New York: John Wiley & Sons.

Bowlby, C. (1993). *Therapeutic activities with persons disabled by Alzheimer's disease and related disorders.* Gaithersburg, MD: Aspen Publishers.

Brawley, E. (1997). *Designing for Alzheimer's disease: Strategies for creating better care environments.* New York: John Wiley & Sons.

Calkins, M.P. (1988). *Design for dementia: Planning environments for the elderly and the confused.* Owings Mills, MD: National Health Press. (Available from I.D.E.A.S., Inc., 440-256–1880)

Calkins, M.P. (1991). *Speaking of weather . . . or isn't there anything else to talk about.* Unpublished paper.

Calkins, M.P. (1995). Homelike is more than carpeting and chintz. *Nursing Homes, 44*(6), 20, 22–25.

Cantril, H. (1978). The human design. In S. Kaplan & R. Kaplan (Eds.), *Humanscape: Environments for people* (pp. 94–101). Ann Arbor, MI: Ulrich's Books.

Cohen, U., & Weisman, G.D. (1991). *Holding on to home: Designing environments for people with dementia.* Baltimore: The Johns Hopkins University Press.

Coons, D.H. (1985). Alive and well at Wesley Hall. *Quarterly, 21*(2), 10–14.

Coons, D.H. (1991). The therapeutic milieu: concepts and criteria. In D.H. Coons (Ed.), *Specialized dementia care units* (pp. 7–24). Baltimore: The Johns Hopkins University Press.

Coons, D., & Spencer B. (1983). The older person's response to therapy: The in-hospital therapeutic community. *Psychiatric Quarterly, 55*(2 & 3), 156–172.

Cooper, C. (1974). The house as symbol of the self. In J.D. Lang, C. Burnette, W. Moleski, & D. Vachon (Eds.), *Designing for human behavior:*

Architecture and the behavioral sciences (pp. 130–146). Stroudsberg, PA: Dowden, Hutchinson & Ross.

Csikszentmihalyi, M., & Rochberg-Halton, E. (1981). *The meaning of things: Domestic symbols and the self.* New York: Cambridge University Press.

Deasy, C.M., & Lasswell, T.E. (1990). *Designing places for people: A handbook on human behavior for architects, designers, and facility managers.* New York: Whitney Library of Design.

Edney, J.J. (1975). Territoriality and control: A field experiment. *Journal of Personality and Social Psychology, 31*(6), 1108–1115.

Emlet, C.A., Crabtree, J.L., Condon, V.A., & Treml, L.A. (1996). *In-home assessment of older adults: An interdisciplinary approach.* Gaithersburg, MD: Aspen Publishers.

Feil, N. (1999). *The validation training program.* Baltimore: Health Professions Press.

Gifford, R. (1997). *Environmental psychology: Principles and practice* (2nd ed.). Boston: Allyn & Bacon.

Glass, D. (1977). Stress, behavior patterns, and coronary disease. *American Scientist, 65,* 177–187.

Goffman, E. (1956). *Presentation of self in everyday life.* New York: Doubleday.

Goffman, E. (1961). *Asylums: Essays on the social situation of mental patients and other inmates.* Garden City, NY: Anchor Books.

Gwyther, L.P. (1985). *Care of Alzheimer's patients: A manual for nursing home staff.* Durham, NC: American Health Care Association and Alzheimer's Disease and Related Disorders Association.

Hellen, C.R. (1992). *Alzheimer's disease: Activity-focused care.* Boston: Andover Medical Publishers.

Hofland, B.F., & David, D. (1990). Autonomy and long-term-care practice: Conclusions and next steps. *Generations,* pp. S91–S94.

Hummon, D. (1989). House, home, and identity in contemporary American culture. In S.M. Low & E. Chambers (Eds.), *Housing, culture, and design* (pp. 207–228). Philadelphia: The University of Pennsylvania Press.

Kane, R.A., Freeman, I.C., Caplan, A.L., Aroskar, M.A., & Urv-Wong, E.K. (1990). Everyday autonomy in nursing homes. *Generations,* pp. S69–S71.

Kaplan, S. (1983). A model of person-environment compatibility. *Environment and Behavior, 15*(3), 311–332.

Kimmel, D.C. (1990). *Adulthood and aging: An interdisciplinary, developmental view* (3rd ed.). New York: John Wiley & Sons.

Krupat, E. (1983). A place for place identity. *Journal of Environmental Psychology, 3,* 343–344.

Magliocco, J.S. (1997). Therapeutic activities for low functioning older adults with dementia. In C.R. Kovach (Ed.), *Late-stage dementia care: A basic guide* (pp. 157–168). London: Taylor & Francis.

Marsden, J.P. (1993). *The architecture of assisted living: Achieving the meanings of home.* Master's thesis, University of Arizona, Tucson.

Miller, D., & Lieberman, M. (1965). The relationship of affect state and adaptive capacity to reactions to stress. *Journal of Gerontology, 20,* 49.

Nissenboim, S., & Vroman, C. (1997). *The positive interactions program of activities for people with Alzheimer's disease.* Baltimore: Health Professions Press.

Omnibus Budget Reconciliation Act of 1987, PL 100-203, § 2, 101 Stat. 1330.

Pinet, C. (1985). *Institutionalized elderly and control over their environment.* Unpublished paper, University of Wisconsin, Milwaukee.

Proffitt, M.A. (1993). *A catalyst for community in sheltered care environments for the elderly: The role of first, second and third place.* Master's thesis, University of Wisconsin, Milwaukee.

Rodin, J. (1986). Aging and health: Effects of the sense of control. *Science, 233,* 1271–1276.

Schulz, R. (1976). Effects of control and predictability on the psychological well-being of the institutionalized aged. *Journal of Personality and Social Psychology, 33,* 563–573.

Seligman, M.E.P. (1975). *Helplessness.* San Francisco: W.H. Freeman.

Sommer, R. (1966). Man's proximate environment. *Journal of Social Issues, 22,* 59–69.

Thomas, W. (1996). *Life worth living: How someone you love can still enjoy life in a nursing home: The Eden Alternative in action.* Acton, MA: VanderWyk & Burnham.

Tobin, S.S. (1996, Fall). Cherished possessions: The meaning of things. *Generations,* pp. 46–48.

Vickery, K. (1998, May). Caregiving east and west of Eden. *Provider,* pp. 89–92, 93–96, 99, 101.

Walsh, M.A. (1990, March). Home sweet homes. *Health Progress,* pp. 35–38.

Wise, K. (1996). Making the choice to carpet. *Nursing Homes Long-Term Care Management, 45*(7), 17–20.

Zavotka, S.L., & Teaford, M.H. (1998, January/February). Design of the public spaces: Does it matter what the lobby looks like? *Ohio Assisted Living Update.*

Zeisel, J., & Tyson, M. (1999). Alzheimer's treatment gardens. In C. Cooper Marcus & M. Barnes (Eds.), *Healing gardens* (pp. 437–504). New York: John Wiley & Sons.

Zgola, J.M. (1987). *Doing things: A guide to programming activities for persons with Alzheimer's disease and related disorders.* Baltimore: The Johns Hopkins University Press.

Zgola, J. (1990). Therapeutic activity. In N.L. Mace (Ed.), *Dementia care: Patient, family, and community.* Baltimore: The Johns Hopkins University Press.

Zgola, J.M., & Bordillon, G. (2001). *Bon appetit! The joy of dining in long-term care.* Baltimore: Health Professions Press.

Appendix A
Resident's
Social
History

The Life of _____

Nickname: _____

Resident's birthdate: _____

Resident's birthplace: _____

First language spoken: _____

Other languages: _____

Mother's name: _____

Mother's occupation: _____

Mother's birthplace: _____

Father's name: _____

Father's occupation: _____

Father's birthplace: _____

Either parent living: _____ Where: _____

Name of person completing this form: _____

Your relationship to resident: _____

Your address: _____

Your telephone number: _____

Describe resident's work history: _____

_____

_____

_____

_____

_____

_____

_____

_____

_____

_____

List resident's past and present social, cultural, civic, volunteer, and other affiliations: _____

_____

_____

_____

_____

_____

_____

_____

List locations where resident has lived: _____

_____

_____

_____

_____

_____

Siblings' names: _____

_____

_____

_____

_____

Siblings living: _____   Where: _____

List most significant family members (e.g., siblings, aunts, best friends, pets) during childhood: _____

_____

_____

_____

Adulthood: _____
_____
_____
_____
_____

Life with Partner

Partner's name: _____

Partner's birthplace: _____

Partner living: _____ Where: _____

If deceased, when: _____

Age when they met: _____

Describe partner and relationship with resident: _____
_____

Wedding date: _____ Where: _____

Most memorable experience as a couple: _____
_____

Number of children: _____

At what age was resident when first child born: _____

Children's names: _____

Grandchildren's names: _____

Some cultural holidays and traditions observed by family: _____
_____

Total number of years resident and partner spent together: _____

Resident's Personality

Which achievements has resident been most proud? _____
_____
_____
_____

Since the onset of dementia, what seems to make the resident most proud:
_____
_____

_____

_____

What have been the resident's greatest strengths in dealing with dementia:

_____

_____

_____

_____

What have been the resident's greatest difficulties in dealing with dementia:

_____

_____

_____

_____

Describe the resident's past crises and his or her methods of coping with them: _____

_____

_____

_____

_____

What seems to bring the resident the most pleasure since the onset of dementia: _____

_____

_____

_____

_____

What has resident traditionally found most relaxing: _____

_____

_____

_____

_____

Since the onset of dementia, what seems to relax the resident most: _____

_____

_____

_____

_____

Describe the resident's typical day: _____

_____

_____

_____

_____

_____

In which of the following roles has the resident traditionally seemed the most comfortable? Circle as many as you like.

parent	boy
child	girl
supervisor	friend
employee	brother
teacher	sister
student	counselor
leader	other: _____
follower	_____
man	_____
woman	_____

Which of the following words best describes the resident's traditional personality? Circle as many as you like.

passive	petty
aggressive	friendly
introverted	reclusive
extroverted	private
demanding	open
conciliatory	controlling
patient	submissive
hot-tempered	gentle
generous	gruff

diligent	humble
careless	nervous
critical	calm
forgiving	other: _____
self-centered	_____
altruistic	_____
proud	_____

Which of the following words best describes the resident's personality since the onset of dementia? Circle as many as you like.

passive	gruff
aggressive	diligent
introverted	careless
extroverted	critical
demanding	forgiving
conciliatory	self-centered
patient	altruistic
hot-tempered	proud
generous	humble
petty	nervous
friendly	calm
reclusive	other: _____
private	_____
open	_____
controlling	_____
submissive	_____
gentle	_____

List every person with whom the resident is in contact weekly or more often.

Name	Relationship (e.g., daughter, friend)	Typical contact (e.g., telephone, letter)

Resident's Leisure Interests

	Participated in	
Active Entertainment	Before dementia	Currently
Bingo	_____	_____
Cards (bridge, poker)	_____	_____
Checkers	_____	_____
Chess	_____	_____
Games (e.g., Scrabble)	_____	_____
Parties	_____	_____
Picnics	_____	_____
Puzzles	_____	_____
Scouting	_____	_____
Service groups	_____	_____
Social clubs	_____	_____
Visits from children	_____	_____
Visits from family	_____	_____
Visits from friends	_____	_____
Volunteering	_____	_____
Other: _____		

_____

	Participated in	
Passive Entertainment	Before dementia	Currently
Listening to radio/favorite programs:		
_____	_____	_____
Reading books, magazines/type: _____	_____	_____
Watching movies/type: _____	_____	_____
Watching TV shows/type:_____	_____	_____
Other: _____		

	Participated in	
Hobbies	Before dementia	Currently
Camping	_____	_____
Ceramics	_____	_____
Dramatics	_____	_____
Driving	_____	_____
Gardening	_____	_____
Home decorating	_____	_____
Leatherwork	_____	_____
Model building	_____	_____
Mosaics	_____	_____
Painting	_____	_____
Photography	_____	_____
Sketching	_____	_____
Traveling	_____	_____
Woodworking	_____	_____
Other: _____		

Home Activities

Cooking	_____	_____
Correspondence	_____	_____
Dusting	_____	_____
Home repairs	_____	_____
Knitting	_____	_____
Laundry	_____	_____
Mending	_____	_____
Mopping	_____	_____
Needlework	_____	_____
Sewing	_____	_____
Shopping	_____	_____
Sweeping	_____	_____
Other: _____		

	Participated in	
Musical Interests	Before dementia	Currently
Attending concerts/type: _____	_____	_____
Playing musical instrument/type: _____	_____	_____
Playing records/type: _____	_____	_____
Radio/TV programs/type: _____	_____	_____
Singing/type of music: _____	_____	_____
Other: _____		

Special Interest Topics	Participated in	
	Before dementia	Currently
Art	_____	_____
Cars	_____	_____
Debates	_____	_____
Fashion	_____	_____
History	_____	_____
Math	_____	_____
Music	_____	_____
Politics	_____	_____
Religion	_____	_____
Science	_____	_____
Social studies	_____	_____
Theater	_____	_____
Travel	_____	_____
Other: _____		

Sports	Participated in	
	Before dementia	Currently
Baseball	_____	_____
Basketball	_____	_____
Billiards	_____	_____
Boating	_____	_____
Bowling	_____	_____
Exercise	_____	_____
Fishing	_____	_____
Football	_____	_____
Golf	_____	_____
Hockey	_____	_____
Horseback riding	_____	_____
Martial arts	_____	_____
Ping pong	_____	_____
Shuffleboard	_____	_____
Soccer	_____	_____
Swimming	_____	_____
Tennis	_____	_____
Volleyball	_____	_____
Walking	_____	_____
Other: _____		

Foods

Likes: _____

_____

_____

_____

_____

Dislikes: _____

_____

_____

_____

_____

Resident's Housing History

Childhood Home (check all that apply)

  — Single family home   — Apartment
  — Duplex   — Rowhouse
  — Mobile home/trailer   — Boarding house
  — Farmhouse   — Other

Location of Childhood Home (check all that apply)

  — Urban   — Suburban   — Rural

State: _____ Country: _____

Previous (most recent) Adult Home (check one)

  — Single family home   — Mobile home/trailer
  — Duplex   — Rowhouse
  — Boarding house   — Condominium
  — Farmhouse   — Other
  — Apartment

Location of Previous (most recent) Adult Home (check one)

  — Urban   — Suburban   — Rural

State: _____ Country: _____

Which of the following words best describes how the resident maintained his/her previous home? (Circle all that apply)

Neat   Messy
Orderly   Clean
Cluttered   Sparse

Which of the following words best describes the previous housing situation of the resident? (Circle all that apply)

Noisy	Dark
Bustling	Quiet
Enclosed	Spacious
Crowded	Bright
Private	

How many people did the resident live with in his or her previous home?___

Which of the following best describes the decor of the resident's previous home? (Circle all that apply)

Traditional	Antiques
Coordinated/matching	Country
Informal	Formal
Contemporary	Other: _____
Eclectic	

What colors were used in the resident's previous home? (Circle all that apply)

Blue	Pink
Orange	Red
Brown	Gold
Purple	White
Green	Peach
Yellow	Other: _____
Beige	

List five home furnishings and/or personal possessions that are most important to the resident and the reasons for their importance.

1. _____

2. _____

3. _____

4. _____

5. _____

Which of the following best describes the vegetation and accessories the resident had in his or her previous garden? (Circle all that apply)

Vegetables	Swings
Trees	Birdbath
Gazebo	Flowers
Birdfeeder	Rocks
Herbs	Rocking chairs
Shrubs	Pond

Approximately how many hours per week did the resident garden or spend time in his or her garden? _____

Appendix B
Hanging Pictures and Artwork

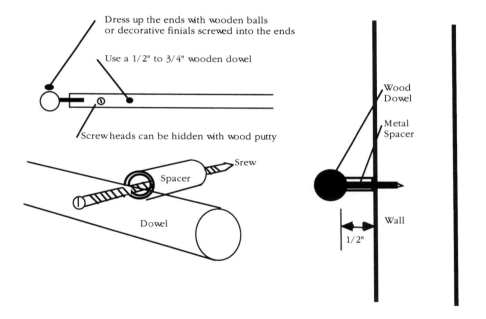

Dress up the ends with wooden balls or decorative finials screwed into the ends

Use a 1/2" to 3/4" wooden dowel

Screw heads can be hidden with wood putty

Srew

Spacer

Dowel

Wood Dowel

Metal Spacer

Wall

1/2"

CREATE YOUR OWN PICTURE HANGING ROD

A picture hanging rod can be made by purchasing a ½- to ¾-inch diameter wood dowel at any hardware or craft store. Decorative end caps such as wood balls or decorative finials usually can be found to screw on to each end. These dowels can be fastened to the wall with modified drapery hangers or screws with spacers. The space between the rod and the wall should be less than

½ inch to keep the pictures stable. Also, decorative drapery rods systems can be modified to attach them to the wall. The cost varies depending on the system.

Mount the dowels to the wall using long screws with ½-inch spacers. (Spacers are metal tubes that should be placed between the wall and the dowel to maintain a fixed distance. This distance should be ½ inch or less to keep pictures from swinging freely.) Screws should be long enough to go through the dowels and should penetrate about ¾ inch into the wall. Make sure the screws are attached to a stud or use appropriate wall anchors. The rods should be supported at least every 2 feet. All holes in the dowel should be predrilled to prevent the wood from splitting.

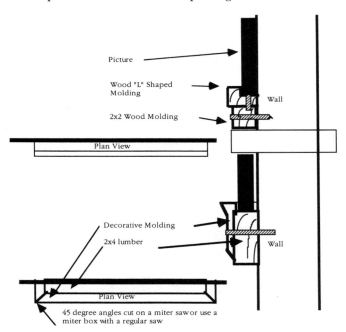

CREATE YOUR OWN PICTURE SHELF

L-shaped moldings (top) can be purchased at any hardware store at a specific cost per linear foot. Small moldings may require a 2-inch by 2-inch molding below to form a shelf on which to fasten the L-shaped wood. For a more decorative (bottom) or substantial look, cove moldings can be cut with a miter saw or miter box at a 45° angle and fastened to a 2-inch by 4-inch board on three sides. Irregular cuts and nail and screw heads can be covered over easily with wood putty. Designs can be as fancy or plain as you prefer. Material costs should be less than $20 for a 4-foot length. Premade shelves also can be purchased for about $45 for a 4-foot length.

Appendix C

Toxicity of Common House and Garden Plants

Potentially Lethal Plants

Common name	Dangerous plant parts	Symptoms
Anemone	Varies by species, but generally entire plant	Severe irritation and blistering of the mucous membranes; if swallowed, causes internal bleeding
Apple	Seed	Abdominal pain, vomiting, lethargy, sweating, coma, and convulsions; large quantities can cause cyanide poisoning
Apricot	Wilted leaves, broken twigs, broken fruit pits	Cyanide poisoning, abdominal pain, vomiting, lethargy, sweating, coma, and convulsions
Autumn crocus	Entire plant, especially seeds and bulbs	Burning of the mouth and throat, intense thirst, nausea, vomiting, and severe diarrhea; occasional involvement of kidneys and dehydration is a danger
Bean tree	Entire plant, especially fruit	Rapid onset of vomiting, drowsiness, weakness, incoordination, sweating, pallor, headaches, and tachycardia
Belladonna	Entire plant but berries are extremely dangerous	Dry mouth, voice loss, tachycardia, elevated temperature, and blurred vision; also causes the inability to pass urine
Black cherry	Wilted leaves, broken twigs, broken fruit pits	Cyanide poisoning, abdominal pain, vomiting, lethargy, sweating, coma, and convulsions
Bleeding heart	Entire plant	Fatal in large quantities, but causes temporary comalike states and labored breathing or convulsions
Burning bush	Entire plant	Delayed onset of symptoms, including diarrhea, persistent vomiting, and convulsions
California privet	Leaves and berries	Colic, vomiting, diarrhea, gastroenteritis, and dehydration
Californian allspice	Seed	Convulsions, myocardial depression, and hypotension
Canadian yew	Foliage, broken seed and bark, although toxicity varies for each plant	Dizziness and dry mouth within 1 hour, then abdominal cramps, salivation, vomiting, rash, causes face to pale, blue lips, weakness, heart arrhythmia, hypotension, and cardiac or respiratory failure
Cardinal flower	Entire plant	Rapid onset of vomiting, drowsiness, weakness, incoordination, sweating, pallor, headaches, and tachycardia
Carolina allspice	Seed	Convulsions, myocardial depression, and hypotension
Castor bean plant	Entire plant, especially seed (1 can kill a small child)	Delayed onset of symptoms, including nausea, vomiting, diarrhea, dehydration, and intestinal dysfunction
Celandine	Entire plant; produces acrid juice	Depression of parasympathetic systems

Plant	Toxic Part	Symptoms
Cherry laurel	Wilted leaves, broken twigs, broken fruit pits	Cyanide poisoning, abdominal pain, vomiting, lethargy, sweating, coma, and convulsions
Chinaberry	Entire plant	Delayed onset of symptoms, including fainting, ataxia, mental confusion, intense gastritis, and vomiting and diarrhea leading to shock; labored respiration, convulsions, paralysis, fatty degeneration of the liver, and kidney damage
Christmas rose	Entire plant	Heart arrhythmia
Clematis	Varies by species, but generally entire plant	Irritation and blistering of skin and mucous membranes, salivation, bloody vomiting and diarrhea, abdominal cramps, dizziness, and convulsions
Common foxglove	Flowers, leaves, and seeds	Affects the heart rate and causes pain, nausea, vomiting, cramps, diarrhea, and convulsions
Common privet	Leaves and berries	Colic, vomiting, diarrhea, gastroenteritis, and dehydration
Crocus	Entire plant, especially seeds and bulbs	Burning of the mouth and throat; intense thirst, nausea, vomiting, and severe diarrhea; occasional involvement of kidneys and dehydration is a danger
Cuckoo-pint	Entire plant	Colorful orange berries may cause esophageal swelling; calcium oxalates cause irritation and swelling of mouth and throat; if eaten, it can cause impaired blood clotting, vomiting, and diarrhea
Daffodil	Bulbs in large quantities	Nausea, persistent vomiting, diarrhea, and dehydration
Daphne	Entire plant, especially fruit	Blistering and swelling of lips, mouth, and throat; salivation; thirst; abdominal pain; vomiting; bloody diarrhea; and loss of electrolytes; may cause kidney damage
Dwarf laurel	Entire plant (even small amounts of leaves may be fatal)	Transient mouth burning; after a few hours, salivation, diarrhea, vomiting, prickling of skin, headaches, severe hypotension, coma, and convulsions
English laurel	Wilted leaves, broken twigs, broken fruit pits	Cyanide poisoning, abdominal pain, vomiting, lethargy, sweating, coma, and convulsions
European spindle tree	Entire plant	Delayed onset of symptoms, including watery diarrhea, persistent vomiting, fever, hallucinations, somnolence, coma, and convulsions

(continued)

165

Potentially Lethal Plants   *(Continued)*

Common name	Dangerous plant parts	Symptoms
False hellebore	Entire plant (fatal only in large quantities)	Cardiac symptoms, burning sensation and pain in upper abdomen, salivation, nausea, vomiting, sweating, blurred vision, and confusion—feels like a heart attack
Fetterbush	Leaves and nectar	Transient mouth burning; hours later, causes salivation, diarrhea, vomiting, prickling of skin, headaches, severe hypotension, coma, and convulsions
Golden chain	Entire plant, especially fruit	Rapid onset of vomiting, drowsiness, weakness, incoordination, sweating, pallor, headaches, and tachycardia
Great lobelia	Entire plant	Rapid onset of vomiting, drowsiness, weakness, incoordination, sweating, pallor, headaches, and tachycardia
Honeysuckle	Varies by species, berries	Severe and persistent vomiting, colic, diarrhea, shock, cardiac arrhythmia, twitching, convulsions, and respiratory failure
Horse chestnut	Young shoots, leaves, flowers, and mature nuts	Severe gastroenteritis leading to electrolyte imbalance; usually fatal after multiple exposures
Huckleberry	Leaves and nectar	Brief burning of mouth; hours later, causes salivation, vomiting, diarrhea, prickling sensation, headaches, weakness, diminished vision, hypotension, coma, and convulsions.
Hydrangea	Flower buds	Cyanide poisoning, abdominal pain, vomiting, lethargy, sweating, coma, and convulsions
Indian tobacco	Entire plant	Rapid onset of vomiting, drowsiness, weakness, incoordination, sweating, pallor, headaches, and tachycardia
Japanese pieris	Leaves and nectar	Transient mouth burning; hours later, causes salivation, diarrhea, vomiting, prickling of skin, headaches, severe hypotension, coma, and convulsions
Japanese skimmia	Entire plant, the red fruit is the usual cause of poisoning	Cardiac arrest
Japanese yew	Foliage, broken seed and bark, although toxicity varies for each plant	Dizziness and dry mouth within 1 hour, then abdominal cramps, salivation, vomiting, rash, causes face to pale, blue lips, weakness, heart arrhythmia, hypotension, and cardiac or respiratory failure
Larkspur	Varies by species, but generally young leaves and seeds	Gastroenteritis, dysfunction of the nervous system

Plant	Toxic part	Symptoms
Lily-of-the-valley	Entire plant	Rash, heart arrhythmia, and gastrointestinal distress; could kill someone with a heart problem
May apple	Entire plant and plant resin except the ripe fruit	Vomiting, intense diarrhea, coma, and kidney failure
Mole plant	Seeds, milky juice is an extreme irritant	Corrosive to membranes and skin, causes acute gastritis
Monkshood	Entire plant	Cardiac arrhythmia; speech difficulties; salivation; nausea; visual blurring; tingling and burning of the lips, tongue, mouth and throat, followed by numbness and constriction
Moonseed	Fruit in large quantities	Convulsions
Mountain laurel	Entire plant (even small amounts of leaves may be fatal)	Transient mouth burning; after a few hours, salivation, diarrhea, vomiting, prickling of skin, headaches, severe hypotension, coma, and convulsions
Mountain tobacco	Flowers and roots	Causes hemorrhage, prostration, chills, and body aches
Oleander	Entire plant	Mouth pain, nausea, vomiting, abdominal pain, cramps, diarrhea, and heart attack
Poppy	Unripe seed capsules	Narcotic overdose, depression of parasympathetic systems
Peach	Wilted leaves, broken twigs, broken fruit pits	Cyanide poisoning, abdominal pain, vomiting, lethargy, sweating, coma, and convulsions
Pernettya	Leaves and nectar	Transient mouth burning; hours later, causes salivation, diarrhea, vomiting, prickling of skin, headaches, severe hypotension, coma, and convulsions
Pin cherry	Wilted leaves, broken twigs, broken fruit pits	Cyanide poisoning, abdominal pain, vomiting, lethargy, sweating, coma, and convulsions
Pokeweed	Older leaves and fruit, but roots are the most dangerous part	Delayed onset of symptoms, including nausea, cramps, profuse sweating, persistent vomiting, diarrhea, and dehydration
Rhododendron	Entire plant, including the nectar	Transient mouth burning; hours later, salivation, diarrhea, vomiting, prickling of skin, headaches, severe hypotension, coma, and convulsions
Rhubarb	Leaves	Extreme diarrhea and kidney failure due to oxalates

(continued)

Potentially Lethal Plants (Continued)

Common name	Dangerous plant parts	Symptoms
Spring meadow saffron	Entire plant, especially seeds and bulbs	Burning of the mouth and throat, intense thirst, nausea, vomiting, and severe diarrhea; occasional involvement of kidneys and dehydration is a danger
Strawberry bush	Entire plant	Delayed onset of symptoms, including diarrhea, persistent vomiting, and convulsions
Sweet bells	Leaves and honey from nectar	Brief burning of mouth; hours later, salivation, vomiting, diarrhea, prickling of skin, headaches, weakness, diminished vision, hypotension, coma, and convulsions
Sweet cherry	Wilted leaves, broken twigs, broken fruit pits	Cyanide poisoning, abdominal pain, vomiting, lethargy, sweating, coma, and convulsions
Sweetshrub	Seed	Convulsions, myocardial depression, and hypotension
Tobacco	Leaves and flowers	Salivation, vomiting, sweating sensation, sensory disorders, convulsions, and vasomotor collapse (breathing stops)
Tree tobacco	Leaves and flowers	Salivation, vomiting, sweating sensation, sensory disorders, convulsions, and vasomotor collapse (breathing stops)
Virginia creeper	Fruit	Severe gastroenteritis
Yew	Foliage, broken seed, and bark, although toxicity varies for each plant	Dizziness and dry mouth within 1 hour, then abdominal cramps, salivation, vomiting, rash, causes face to pale, blue lips, weakness, heart arrhythmia, hypotension, and cardiac or respiratory failure

Rarely Fatal Plants

American bittersweet	Flowers, leaves, and seeds	Vomiting, diarrhea
Anemone	Varies by species, but generally entire plant	Severe irritation and blistering of the mucous membranes; if swallowed, causes internal bleeding
Black locust	Inner bark, seeds and young leaves	Delayed onset of symptoms, including nausea, vomiting, and diarrhea
Bleeding heart	Entire plant	Fatal in large quantities; temporary comalike states, labored breathing or convulsions
Bog rosemary	Entire plant	Gastric upset

Boxwood	Leaves and twigs	Nervous symptoms, vomiting
Buttercup	Entire plant	Gastrointestinal distress, burning and blistering of all mucous membranes, lips, and mouth
Calla lily	Stems, leaves (if chewed)	Extreme tongue swelling, intense burning of lips and mouth
Chinese wisteria	Entire plant	Abdominal pain, nausea, vomiting
Dragonroot	Rhizomes	Severe irritation if chewed
Elderberry	Entire plant except cooked ripe berries	Although small amounts of raw, black fruit may be eaten, plant can cause mild to severe diarrhea
English ivy	Berries and leaves	Throat burning, sometimes gastrointestinal distress
European beech	Seed	Reactions vary, depending on the person
Four-o'clocks	Nuts and seeds	Stomach pain, vomiting
Holly	Berries	Nausea, vomiting, diarrhea
Hyacinth bean	Raw seed	Gastrointestinal distress and lots of gas; cooked beans are nontoxic
Hyacinth	Bulbs	Severe upset stomach
Iris	Varies by species, but generally entire plant	Gastrointestinal irritant
Japanese aucuba	Fruit	Vomiting, fever
Japanese wisteria	Entire plant	Abdominal pain, nausea, vomiting
Kentucky coffee tree	Seed and pulp between seed	Nausea, sweating, is a mild form of nicotine poisoning
Lily-of-the-valley	Entire plant	Rash, heart arrhythmia, and gastrointestinal distress; could kill someone with a heart problem
Lupine	Leaves and seeds	Hallucinations
Marsh marigold	Older plant parts	Acute inflammation and mouth blistering; if swallowed, causes bloody diarrhea, vomiting.
Matrimony vine	Entire plant	Gastrointestinal upset
Morning glory	Seed and roots	Visual and neural disturbances; some people react violently enough to be hospitalized
Oak	Raw acorns	Binds with calcium in body and can cause calcium deficiency in blood, leading to heart irregularity; raw acorns have high amounts of tannin, which is implicated in esophageal cancers
Red mulberry	Overripe fruit and milky sap	Digestive and nervous upset

(continued)

Rarely Fatal Plants *(Continued)*

Common name	Dangerous plant parts	Symptoms
Scotch broom	Entire plant, especially seed	There may be no immediate symptoms, but there are carcinogens in the plant and some slow-acting alkaloids
Shoo-fly plant	Leaves and berries	Nausea, vomiting, depression
Snowdrop	Bulbs	Vomiting, diarrhea
Spring adonis	Entire plant	Mouth and stomach irritation
Squill	Entire plant, especially bulbs	Delayed onset of symptoms, including mouth pain, nausea, vomiting abdominal pain, cramps, diarrhea, and possible heart arrhythmia
Star-of-Bethlehem	Flower and bulbs	Mouth pain, nausea, vomiting, stomach pain, cramps
Summer pheasant's eye	Entire plant	Mouth and stomach irritation
Sweet pea	Seeds	Would have to be eaten in large quantities, but causes temporary paralysis
Thorn apple	Entire plant	Severe disorientation, manic states

From American Nursery Magazine. (April 15, 1996). *Potentially lethal plants*. Chicago: American Nurseryman; reprinted by permission.

Index

Page numbers followed by *f* indicate figures; those followed by *t* indicate tables. This is a comprehensive index covering Volumes 1–4 of *Creating Successful Dementia Care Settings*. The first number of each entry indicates the volume; the second number indicates the page.

ORDER THESE COMPANION VIDEOS FOR CREATING SUCCESSFUL DEMENTIA CARE SETTINGS

Video 1
Maximizing Cognitive and Functional Abilities/No. 2769/40-min VHS/$92

Video 2
Minimizing Disruptive Behaviors/No. 2777/21-min VHS/$55

Video 3
Enhancing Self and Sense of Home/No. 2785/33-min VHS/$78

Prices are subject to change.

ORDER FORM

Please send me the following video(s):

Stk No.	Title	Quantity	Price

SHIPPING & HANDLING			
For pre-tax total of	*Add*	Subtotal	
$0.00 to $49.99	$5.00	MD residents, add 5% tax	
$50.00 to $399.99	10%	Shipping & Handling	
$400.00 and over	8%	TOTAL	

❑ Check enclosed (payable to **Health Professions Press**)

❑ Bill my institution (attach purchase order) ❑ MasterCard ❑ Visa ❑ AmEx

Credit card#/Exp. date _____

Signature _____

Name _____

Address _____
(Orders cannot be shipped to P.O. boxes)

City/State/ZIP _____

Daytime phone _____

HEALTH PROFESSIONS PRESS   P.O. BOX 10624   BALTIMORE, MD 21285-0624
TOLL FREE (888) 337-8808   FAX (410) 337-8539
www.healthpropress.com

ZCK